To Amanda
Best wishes
Evelyn.

"Life Beyond The Waistline"
the expanding role of an NHS dietitian

GW00357623

e Beyond the Waistline

The Expanding Role of an NHS Dietitian

Evelyn Newman

Overview

Evelyn is a multi-award-winning retired dietitian who has worked in a wide variety of roles and locations across the UK over four decades. She is well known to colleagues across the UK and has been a regular contributor to many national publications, on-line platforms and events. She has also volunteered for the British Dietetic Association (BDA) in a variety of roles since 1987. Her career path is unique to anyone in the profession and has taken her to work in places that no one could have imagined employing a dietitian when she started her student journey back in 1982. Her experience as a dietitian is certainly not the stereotypical characterisation that one might imagine and there is very little reference to people trying to lose weight – hence the title of the book. This is an autobiographical memoir, full of insights, stories, anecdotes and reflections of the many experiences her roles have offered and the people she has worked alongside in so many environments. Evelyn has seen many changes to dietetic practice, the profession and the NHS over the years but has always embraced and enjoyed these, readily taking on many new opportunities and challenges ahead of any other UK dietitian. Her positive outlook on life has helped in her personal and professional development, promoting the role of dietitians in many diverse settings, such as the prison service, football clubs, regional renal and burns units, the TUC and Whitehall. She has won several national awards and been selected to present her transformational work, sharing with colleagues in many international venues and events. The book takes readers on her journeys to New York state correctional facilities, a tour of Indian burns units, across to Europe, to Northern Ireland, Iceland and to the many towns and cities where she's worked over the years. It is a story of perseverance, thankfulness, success and encouragement for others to be open to all possibilities.

Introduction

They say that you know you're getting old when you start thinking about the old days. Well, I found myself doing just that a few years ago, even though, in my head, I'll always think of myself as a young 36.

I initially started thinking about writing this book around the 70th anniversary of the NHS, having written an article reflecting on how my career had developed over the many years since leaving university. It was published in both the Scottish press and on a Scottish government blog site, which went out widely on Twitter, resulting in lots of really positive comments from a variety people both in and outside of work. Many NHS colleagues and acquaintances were surprised to hear how uniquely varied my roles had been and a few quipped that I should write a book about my experiences because they were so different to the public perception of what a dietitian did. The stereotype is, of course, of someone who either helps obese people to lose weight or is some kind of a muesli-munching veggie who frowns on anyone eating an unhealthy diet. Both generalisations are, thankfully, incorrect and in my case, they are way off the mark. I have been very fortunate to be able to steer a career course that bucked the trend of conventional dietetics, allowing me to move around the country, changing roles and areas of specialist interest. I have also been able to maximise the many unusual opportunities that came my way, taking me to places I would otherwise never have dreamed of getting to.

My upbringing in the Northeast of Scotland gave no indication of what I might go onto achieve, being the eldest of three siblings in a one-parent family, which was heavily reliant on state benefits. There was no expectation that I would do well at school, never mind go to university, but I have always had a strong sense of confidence in my own abilities and was determined to prove to any doubters that they were wrong. That has been a theme of my general approach throughout life and it has enabled me to never feel constrained by others' limited opinions, any self-doubt or the general view of what might be possible. I have a strong work ethic and always believe that anything is possible if you put your mind to it, coupled with a bit of effort. When I hear people saying that something always has to be done a certain way, I see it almost as a challenge to question why that might be and look at how it might be transformed using a more innovative approach.

I am so grateful to the NHS for the many years of employment, variety and opportunity to work with so many groups of staff and members of the public, across so many different care settings. The role of a dietitian has evolved far beyond my expectations and earlier experiences as it has adapted to numerous clinical, professional and service developments. Perhaps my recollections will prompt some to reminisce about their own working life and maybe even enthuse others to take up the baton of innovation and release even greater transformational potential for their future roles and careers. As I settle into an exciting new phase of life in retirement, and the undoubted opportunities that will bring, I hope that you enjoy my story. And if you were part of that story, thank you.

Contents

Overview v

Introduction vii

Chapter 1 — Student life 1

Chapter 2 — Putting it into practice 31

Chapter 3 — The early years 63

Chapter 4 — Burning challenges. 79

Chapter 5 — Moving on................................. 129

Chapter 6 — Onwards and upwards 143

Chapter 7 — Life in the Southeast............... 161

Chapter 8 — Life behind bars 175

Chapter 9 — The cabinet office leadership programme 223

Chapter 10 — Volunteering with the BDA 239

Chapter 11 — Affiliation with the TUC 263

Chapter 12 — A national role......................... 279

Chapter 13 — The Highlands 297

Chapter 14 — New beginnings 325

Chapter 15 — The digital coming of age 355

Chapter 16 — COVID 363

Chapter 17— Retirement 371

Chapter 18 — Reflections 379

Acknowledgements 385

Glossary of terms 387

References 390

Chapter 1 — Student life

I can clearly remember being interviewed for a place at Robert Gordon's Institute of Technology (now Robert Gordon's University – RGU) by the head of school, Dr David Livingstone. I had no idea what to expect from my first-ever interview but to say the experience was informal is an understatement. He was sat back with his feet up on the desk and hands folded over his stomach. I discovered later that he thought this would help to keep students relaxed and that the meeting was more about getting to know us and how well we might fit into life as a student dietitian. My handwritten application was lying on the desk next to him. In those days, we actually had to declare our weight and height, to ensure that no one was accepted onto the course if they potentially had an eating disorder or were very overweight. There was a very clear expectation of how a dietitian should look and it was generally believed that no patient or colleagues could take an obese or anorexic dietitian seriously. Why that should ever have even featured in a decision about anyone's career path is bizarre. I doubt whether the same bias existed for medical students or nurses who didn't look after their health by smoking or drinking too much alcohol.

My one and only careers interview in 6th year had been a revelation to me. I had no real idea what I wanted to do after leaving school, so, when I was asked about the subjects I was studying, the advisor started flicking through a variety of reference magazines and that's where the degree course for nutrition and dietetics appeared. I wasn't sure what I'd be able to do as a dietitian; did it mean just telling people how to lose weight? That was the stereotypical view of the job, which was still a very new profession at the time. Then again, that was part of the appeal, I suppose — being different — but in the end, I thought that anything to do with food would have lots of potential and it turned out that I was right. I never regretted applying for the course or the career path that unfolded in the years ahead.

I waited several weeks before receiving the offer of a place at RGU, conditional on gaining a C or above in Higher biology. I had been brought up in a single-parent household, in council accommodation, heavily reliant on the various social security benefits of the day. Money was always very tight and I was fortunate to have a steady part-time job in a local chemist's shop. However, I was determined to break out of the cycle of poverty, dependence on handouts and hand-me-downs so I put every effort into my studies. After a nail-biting wait for the postman to bring my results in August 1982, a registered letter arrived — no email or text alerts back then! I was thrilled to have the much needed C, which proved all the extra studying had been worth it. I was excited and couldn't wait to get started the much needed degree, which would eventually lead me to so many new places, unbelievable opportunities and a secure future career in the NHS.

I moved through to Aberdeen a couple of days before the start of the course, having rented a room, with one of my friends, in a family house just off Queen's Cross in the west end. Fiona moved out after a year, but I remained with The Peats for the rest of my university studies, only moving out during summer holidays. I continued to keep in touch with my (now late) landlady long afterwards and always felt very fortunate for having had such a nice, warm welcoming place to live and study throughout my time in Aberdeen. The first week of student life was a whirl of form-filling, working out our timetables and trying to navigate where everything was. I met Jan, who has remained my closest friend for all these years, and because our surnames were closest alphabetically, we found ourselves next to each other for most of the practical work sessions. Matriculation cards were produced and student grants were paid to us as individual cheques (no internet banking in those days). All university tuition was free (as it still remains in Scotland) and grants were paid on a means-tested basis. Because of my family circumstances, I received the full grant each term and had more money than I could have ever imagined in my bank. I started to eat much better and enjoyed joining friends for meals out. We started the first day with a list of items that we were expected to buy before lessons started for real the following week: Two white coats — 1 for catering and one for lab work — a large Good Housekeeping cookbook for our soon-to-be infamous cooking sessions, a set of quality kitchen knives, which I still use today, and a variety of textbooks. New clothes soon became a priority as I outgrew everything after the first term, having gained much needed weight and height with a much better personal diet. After three years and a lot of disciplined study, I qualified with a BSc degree in nutrition and dietetics back in 1985. However, it wasn't always plain sailing and I very nearly didn't make it past my first year.

Funnily enough, it was nothing to do with my academic ability. I worked really hard to even be pretty average in subjects as diverse as biochemistry, physics, psychology and microbiology. My Achilles heel was much more practical — catering — and, more particularly, in cooking family meals! The trouble was that cooking for the apparent 'families' we were catering for, we were using food and kitchen equipment that bore no resemblance to any that had ever appeared in my home growing up. When I started at RGU, I was quite underweight and anaemic because of years of relying on government benefits and of eating a very limited poorly balanced diet. Janet Lowell, our catering lecturer, took me aside towards the end of first year to gently explain that I was in danger of not progressing to second year if my performance didn't improve.

This wasn't a surprise to me, or my fellow students, who regularly fell about laughing at my lack of knowledge of raw ingredients and the many mishaps in my food preparation. Each week, it wasn't so much a question of whether I would make a mistake, it was how big and hilarious it would be. I wasn't trying to be funny or deliberately stupid; I just genuinely didn't know what I was doing. Even today, Jan still tells the story of how I managed to turn a recipe for six portions of cold cucumber soup (you see what I mean about family cooking?) into an individual portion complete with a hint of carbon... You guessed it; I left it cooking on the gas stove (I'd never used one before) on too high a heat and neglected to notice that it was slowly evaporating and sticking to the bottom of the pan.

I had managed to get myself distracted with even more confusion about the main course I was assigned to prepare — Turkish three bean salad. The only experience I'd previously had with beans was the popular 57 variety, served with sausages and mash at home. Not only did I have to work out which beans were which, I was panicking because the salad dressing contained fresh herbs, of which I had no previous experience. There was an array of green stalks laid out with other ingredients for the class to select for preparing the different meals we were all assigned to make. When I asked Janet for help identifying some mint, she pointed to a bunch on the table and left me to it. When she returned twenty minutes later, she was clearly confused as I proudly showed off my hard work. She asked where the mint was and it quickly became clear that the leaves, which I'd stripped off and thrown in the waste bin, should have been chopped up and mixed into the salad dressing. Instead, there were small, carefully chopped pieces of mint stalks mixed throughout the dish, making it pretty much inedible! I felt so disappointed in myself— it had been really hard work to cut it up! Suddenly, we were alerted to the distinctive smell of burning coming from the stove…

Through tears of laughter, Jan and Lesley, in the neighbouring cooking stations, called others over to see the catering carnage. Even Janet was finding it hard not to join in. I can only imagine the amusement in the staff room later when she shared yet another afternoon of my catering disasters with her colleagues. It wasn't just ingredients that I struggled with either; I had never used some of the equipment before. At home, I had been the one coming home from school and cooking tea but mainly used the oven, grill and ever-present chip pan, full of lard, in our kitchen. We had no fridge freezer, never mind fancy modern gadgets. So, one day, when I arrived for class to see that I would have to use a food processor, my anxiety levels reached new heights but I was still determined to try and get it right. I was tasked with making mayonnaise from scratch, which involved slowly and carefully adding ingredients to prevent the mixture from separating. Janet approached my workstation with a now familiar expression of curious hopelessness. I couldn't understand why I didn't seem to be getting anywhere, watching the egg yolks whirling round. Why was my mayonnaise not developing? She stepped closer with a hint of a smile quivering at the side of her mouth. Lifting the clear stopper out of the opening in the blender where ingredients should be added, she pointedly handed it to me. Immediately, I realised that I had been adding my mixture into the stopper, which is why the mayonnaise wasn't materialising — what a basic error! As Janet walked off shaking her head, laughter from my classmates erupted around the room once again.

Despite it being a steep learning curve for me, the year really expanded my knowledge and catering repertoire and allowed me to try out so many new dishes and ingredients that I might never otherwise have come across.

Thankfully, I managed to scrape through catering with the lowest pass mark and started to look forward to my next year. However, readers may not be surprised to know that I have never since felt the need to make cold cucumber soup, homemade mayonnaise or Turkish three bean salad...

The course was pretty much full time over 5 days a week back then. We studied sociology, psychology, nutrition science, microbiology, physiology, biochemistry, statistics and physics and I had to work really hard to keep on top of all the new information and assignments. I became very adept at taking copious real-time notes, and today, I can still look ahead at presentations while simultaneously writing in my notepad.

We were a close network of 40 students, coming from a variety of backgrounds and nations: "Poom" was from Thailand, Kitty came from Hong Kong and kept many people entertained with palm reading; there were two students from Kenya who sadly didn't make it into second year; Alison from Armagh in N. Ireland; a variety of people from England; while the rest of us were Scots, including two others from my hometown.

Thankfully, I made it through our many first-year exams and was glad to finally finish my studies of both physics and statistics — the latter being an open-book test, which I just scraped through with the help of other students' notes. 1982 was also the year when I became a student member of the British Dietetic Association (BDA) and enjoyed receiving the monthly printed magazine and associated information that was posted to us. Students weren't allowed to receive the regular jobs list that was sent to full members, so we had to wait to learn more about vacancies from dietitians on placement in later years. I also became elected as a class representative for my year, which was probably where my later love of industrial relations came from.

Looking for work in the summer of 1983 and the following Easter holidays, I became a temporary hospital cleaner. This allowed me to remain financially independent while living in Aberdeen, working in two local elderly care settings — Woodend and Morningfield Hospitals. It gave me a real insight into the hard work that hospital cleaners have to do and a lifelong appreciation for their contribution to the smooth running of all health and social care settings. I had a few challenges using the large, powerful floor buffers, as I was still quite underweight. On one occasion, another cleaner managed to avert a nasty accident when the cable for the machine became wrapped round the buffing pad. It pulled me close to the machine as the cable had been held round my waist and I was struggling to move. She leaned down behind me and switched it off at the wall, giving me a few minutes to slowly extricate myself and calm down before carrying on where I left off. Little did I know how relevant this work, and insights from it, would be many years later when I was interviewed for and appointed to the role of head of nutrition and cleaning for England and Wales!

In September 1983, second year started optimistically but still included catering; this time, though, it was done on a large scale. Our lecturer was a rotund, ginger-bearded ex-RAF chef with many years of experience of bulk catering. The sessions were designed to help us appreciate the challenges of cooking for large numbers, scaling up the weight of ingredients and the size of the equipment. For the most part, I managed better because I was working as part of a small team or in pairs and other students knew much more about ingredients than me, helping to disguise my ignorance of many.

The format of our biochemistry lectures changed in 2nd year as we were joined by pharmacy students for lessons in the city-centre lecture theatres. Chris Fenn became our food science lecturer and made the lessons really interactive, fun and interesting. We continued studying physiology, microbiology, psychology and sociology but studying was more manageable as we had all developed a good routine and encouraged each other lots. All of my classmates were a really nice group of colleagues to be with and if we bumped into each other over the years at various events, we still greeted each other with great friendship and enjoy memories from those times.

Lab work was at the RGU building in the centre of Aberdeen, and the smell of various chemicals lingered in clothes and hair long after we left for the day. At the time, I was very committed to anti-vivisection and approached Dr Livingstone to ask if I could opt out of any actual dissections. He found it somewhat amusing but agreed and I was allowed to observe Jan and Lesley carry out theirs instead. As if my principles might be responsible for saving the short life of a small lab rodent!

At weekends, I would often babysit for a young Mauritian family who were living in the city while the husband worked in a large multi-national oil company. It meant I could study while the two siblings slept and this broke up the routine of the week.

Back in 1983, the second-year dietetic curriculum required us to carry out a catering placement in a commercial large-scale kitchen for 4 weeks during the summer holidays. I ended up working as part of the catering team in the headquarters of a multinational oil company in Aberdeen. The staff were friendly, and I was given opportunities to cook, to work in the office covering for the administrator who was on holiday, and to help front of house, serving the public. While that sounded like something of a promotion, and, in many ways it was, I nearly didn't manage to take up the offer. Since school, I hadn't owned or worn a skirt, and certainly never small heels, and had to make a special trip to town to buy something suitable. The fantastic choice and quality of the food and drinks being served for their lunches were beyond anything that I'd ever come across – those employees were so fortunate. I felt so lucky, knowing that many of my classmates were doing their placements in hospitals, fish processing plants and other less glamorous businesses! I ate really well and thoroughly enjoyed the experience. RGU provided me with accommodation in the city centre for the summer. It was character-building to say the least, sharing a second-floor tenement flat above a butcher's shop. The smell was something to behold in the heatwave that year. I found myself living in a flat with three others and I was sharing a room with a very wild pharmacy student from the Highlands. Unfortunately, she had quite an appetite for Night Nurse and vodka cocktails, which made for some sleepless nights as she stumbled around in the dark ricocheting between my bed and the wardrobe. At every opportunity, I headed back home to Elgin for some respite from the sensory onslaughts of the flat, and for some peace and a good sleep! There were challenges during the catering placement too, of course, but the ones I faced were more to do with the limitations of my size, rather than my knowledge. After all, I've never been either the tallest or strongest of people. On one occasion, I was asked to take through a large platter of rollmop herrings to the front servery and had to stretch forward and upwards on my tiptoes to reach the surface. As I did so, the tray tipped slightly and cold fishy liquid started to run down my arms beneath my kitchen whites. Ever the professional, I didn't let out the piercing scream that was echoing around my head! There were customers around after all and I didn't want to risk it dripping into the lovely selection of puddings and gateaux below. Somehow, I managed to take it down and retreat back to the kitchen where I got Jack, the six-foot-tall head chef, to take it back through for me. The smell stuck with me for the rest of the day though, and I can only imagine what other bus passengers thought of me as I headed home later! During the second week, I was assigned to work with Shona, the pastry chef, making some very high-calorie puddings, using gallons of double cream in an industrial mixer. She was quite a big lady and thought nothing of picking up the steel bowls as they were whisking cake mixtures, manually moving them around to stop it sticking on the sides. One day, while she was talking with Jack, in a moment of sheer madness, I took it upon myself to do the same thing. As soon as the bowl was lifted out of its secure setting, I nearly took off, and in a scene of comic chaos, I had to shout for help. She switched off the machine at the wall and looked long and hard at me as I stood shaking in shock and embarrassment before walking off to continue her conversation. Needless to say, I left the mixing bowl where it should have been and we continued again as if nothing had happened. Despite a few other hilarious hiccups, they actually invited me back to work as a paid employee, which helped fund my summer holiday that year, hitch-hiking around Europe with a school friend. I returned to RGU with tales and photos of my travels and looking tanned and healthier than I'd ever been in my life. Third year also started on a note of sadness as we learned that Anne, one of our fellow students, who came from Penicuik, had succumbed to complications of multiple sclerosis and had passed away over the summer. It was particularly sad for Shirley, her best friend in class, and we all tried to support her as best we could. For many, the year brought a new feeling of personal optimism and possibilities. We were now the oldest of the dietetic students, as the fourth years were all away on their practical hospital placements around the UK. We were introduced to speakers from local hospitals and spent more time on visits to Aberdeen Royal Infirmary. The medical library was a distracting place to study though, as jars of various preserved body parts/organs were displayed around the desk spaces – some of them quite gory. One afternoon, a "real" dietitian even came to talk to us at RGU about life on the hospital wards. That's where we were all expected to end up working, as there was little in the way of variety of career opportunities back then. She stood at the front looking very professional, wearing the standard issue white coat, and had a long thin plastic feeding tube draped round her neck, much like doctors do with a stethoscope. At the time, we were all fascinated and enthused by our glamorous speaker who inspired us all to look forward to the opportunities of working on wards in the future. Those were the very early days of nasogastric tubes and she was telling us about the role of dietitians in calculating tube feeds. The wider bore, more rigid Ryles tubes were still much more commonly used to allow thick, viscous homemade feeds to pass through them. Back then, diet cooks had to prepare them in the diet kitchen, though the numbers of patients receiving them was relatively small compared to the volumes used today. It's hard to believe that raw eggs were used in this way, mixed with milk, double cream and sugar. Patients were also routinely given liquidised soup, cups of tea and other conventional, liquidised food via these wide-bore tubes. Today's clinicians will be horrified to read this but it was all done in the ward kitchens by nursing staff. Over the coming years, narrower, more comfortable and durable polyurethane tubes were developed, which meant that they needed to be changed less often and patients tolerated them better.

Today, we take them for granted, but in the mid-80s, "Silk" tubes (named after the professor who developed them) were very expensive. So, more often than not, wards still used large-bore Ryles tubes and the narrower PVC versions, which still had to be changed every week. The newer tubes had a guide wire to aid insertion and, before it could be used, patients had to be x-rayed to check that they had been correctly positioned in the stomach rather than the lungs, which would have potentially been fatal. It would be several years before we saw polyurethane nasogastric tubes, never mind life-changing gastrostomies and jejunostomies — even then, they were used only very occasionally. It wasn't until we moved into the early 90s that it became more routine practice, but even then, they were only used for people in hospital settings. Home enteral feeding, where patients could care for themselves and operate their own feeding pumps, was still an unthinkable option. It slowly evolved over the years ahead and was a great way of freeing up hospital beds, allowing individuals and their families to have greater independence and autonomy in their own homes, schools and workplaces. It also saw the evolution of more specialist roles for dietitians, reaching out into community settings, raising the profile and perceived value of the profession with GPs and other primary care colleagues. Students today have to be familiar with a far wider range of tubes, buttons, pumps, feeds and services than we did back then when enteral feeding was in its infancy. The first manufactured tube feeds to be used in most hospitals in the 1980s were made by one company with only two varieties — 1kcal/ml or 1.5kcal/ml. They came in a tinned format and were either administered by syringe boluses or had to be decanted into plastic reservoirs before use. For many years afterwards, tube feeds were colloquially referred to as "Clinifeeds" and referrals would arrive in the department for a patient to be "Clinifed". The feeds were usually given over 24 hours, rather than giving the bowel some rest, which we are familiar with now. This resulted in many sleepless nights for patients while nursing staff had to interrupt them to administer the bolus feed during the night. The whole process was made even more uncomfortable if the nurse had taken the tin of feed straight from a fridge or cold store, without first letting it reach room temperature. Syringing chilly fluid down the oesophagus is actually quite an uncomfortable, even painful experience. Nasogastric feeding was the modus operandi of the day but the tubes could be very cumbersome and awkward, hanging out of someone's nose. Often, staff would forget to change them weekly and they could easily become clogged with solid feed. Ward staff used a variety of methods to try and unblock feeding tubes rather than removing them. Some tried a powerful syringeful of water, some fizzy cola, a solution of bicarbonate of soda or even sherry! If that didn't work, the tube would have to come out and be replaced with another one causing further delay until the position of the tube was double-checked. Occasionally, one would find its way into someone's lung, causing a coughing fit, but if the patient was unconscious, it could go unnoticed, causing pneumonia or even death. Tube feeds were also associated with loose stools and ward staff would often call down to departments asking for patients to be reviewed due to "feeding diarrhoea". It was usually nothing to do with the feed. The effects on the bowel from the administration of intravenous antibiotics were more likely to be the cause and were often the reason for putting ward staff off tube-feeding patients back then.

Another new topic for third year at RGU was business studies. None of us were quite sure why we were learning about banking, accountancy and marketing, but, on reflection, I can see that it would have been very useful for anyone considering a role in management or in private practice. The lecturer was a young self-confident guy who seemed to know a lot about technology — a foreign language to most of us back then. I can still remember him telling us about groundbreaking work being developed, which would one day allow people to pay for goods by just using a bank card inserted in a machine or at petrol pumps... Younger readers will now be shaking their heads in disbelief but we really were that far behind compared to life today. At that time, even automated cash machines weren't that common so much of what he was telling us seemed pretty far-fetched. Amusingly, he was totally and hopelessly smitten with "Spike", one of our classmates, and was always looking for ways to bring her into the conversation. We all thought it was hilarious and she generally sat at the back of class, with her friend Susan, to try and avoid him. Much to her annoyance, one afternoon, he took great interest in the fur coat she was wearing and made a big thing of walking forward to take a closer look. He was being very complimentary and was clearly hoping that she would enjoy the attention. He asked her if it was mink. "No," she replied, deadpan, "it's mole!" We all erupted with laughter and he retreated, red-faced to try and regain his composure.

Catering practicals in 3rd year focused entirely on planning and preparing therapeutic diets needed for patients to live well with a variety of medical conditions. This also meant that we had to calculate nutritional composition of the meals we were preparing, manually using our trusty copies of "McCance". Nowadays, nutrition software packages do it all for you but we had to painstakingly handwrite it all longhand and work it all out from scratch, with brainpower and calculators. It formed part of our ongoing assessment over the year, so we took it very seriously and it certainly helped us to build a solid foundation of learning which was very useful to us in our future practice.

We had to hand in our list of ingredients at the start of the week so that they were ready for us in the kitchen each Friday for the 3-hour catering practical. We had to really get to grips with how or whether our dietetic advice might translate into palatability for our patients and that also meant that we had to try out a variety of manufactured, prescribable products. There was a limited range of gluten-free foods available on prescription for people living with coeliac disease: tins of bread, digestive biscuits and some very gelatinous dried spaghetti. The varieties used at the time smelled and tasted quite awful but we experimented a bit and soon learned a few tricks to improve the flavour and texture of some. Worse was to come though, in the form of the early forms of elemental drinks and flavourings for people with digestive absorption disorders. They came in small tins and had separate flavouring sachets which could be mixed with the foul-smelling liquid, in the vain hope that it might taste better— it did not as we discovered when we had to taste them all! We found the best solution was to cover the top of the cup with clingfilm or a lid if possible and take sips using a straw— anything to avoid the smell.

The key role of any dietitian is to translate science into practice but it is so important that we truly understand the impact of restrictive diets and the challenges of being able to follow our advice if the food we recommend is unpalatable. Product ranges— prescribable and retail— have continued to develop to a far higher standard, offering greater variety and improved flavours in many cases. This results in greater patient compliance with their specialist diets, less complications and better management of long term conditions such as coeliac disease, PKU, inflammatory bowel disorders and a whole range of food allergies.

A new nutrition sciences lecturer, Dr Alan Wise, began working with us at the start of term, having moved to Aberdeen from carrying out research work at a University in Iran. He had a very serious demeanour and spoke with a high-pitched squeaky voice, causing lots of amusement to us all. He was, however, the first person to introduce us all to the possibilities of using computers as a way of carrying out nutritional analysis during our one hour of IT per week. Most of us had never even seen a real one and no one had much, if any, experience of what we would be able to use one for when we started work as dietitians. They were confined to one locked room and were as huge as they were basic— for those of you who can remember life before modern programming. They weren't even common in most workplaces so it would be quite a few years before any of us actually had access to one, never mind the software needed to analyse recipes and menus. Letters had to be handwritten before being typed (on an actual typewriter) by department secretaries, if you were fortunate to have one, moving on to the use of manual Dictaphones, so far removed from the digital dictation expected as standard by so many clinicians today.

Dr Colin Henderson was our microbiology lecturer and clearly enjoyed the topic. At one point, he had us all taking swabs and samples from all around the building, including toilet bowls, to grow whatever bugs were there on a wide variety of petri dishes. What he didn't know about a "trickling filter system" wasn't worth knowing!

In February 2005, Jan, me and Jackie— a fellow student— hosted our 21st birthday party at The Amatola Hotel in the west end of Aberdeen. My landlady, Mrs Peat, printed off our tickets and we hired a wonderful Scottish dance band for a great evening packed full of family, friends and fellow students. The Amatola has long since been demolished and turned into modern flats but the memories remain. It was a rite of passage for many of us in our year and strengthened the bonds we had as the class of '85.

In preparation for our final degree exams, we all studied really hard, revising for long hours in the library and at home. One poor girl took it all a bit far though and ended up as a patient in Aberdeen Royal infirmary herself, nearly missing out on the chance to take her exams. She had left her studying a bit late in the term and had attempted to cram her revision by staying awake for many hours by taking caffeine pills.

Naturally, she experienced frightening palpitations and needed close on-ward observation, attached to a heart monitor, before being discharged back home with a stern warning not to try that again.

Chapter 2 — Putting it into practice

During the year, fourth-year students returned to RGU fresh and enthusiastic from their practical placements all over the UK. They had been working alongside "real" dietitians in hospital wards with actual patients and were ready to start applying for jobs themselves. We had the chance to hear about the places they'd worked and the experiences they'd had. I was completely captivated by the stories from Katy, who had spent her time "working" on placement in Bristol. It was hundreds of miles away from my home in the northeast of Scotland, but I was always looking for the chance for adventure and to explore other parts of the country. As our travel and accommodation costs were being paid for us, I thought it would be a great opportunity to see if I could arrange to have my own placement there too. The curriculum for student dietitians back then meant that you had to complete a 32-week practical training programme, covering areas such as catering management, renal dietetics, community practice and general clinical work. A 4-week complimentary placement in another hospital setting also had to be organised within the 32-week period and was designed to give you a different experience in another area of practice. Once all that was finished, you were expected to arrange and successfully complete an eleven-week "industrial" placement for yourself, beyond clinical settings. Some people managed to arrange time in food production companies but opportunities in those days were very limited and many colleagues ended up in different community hospitals, working alongside catering teams. After all that, we were to return to Aberdeen with evidence of our successful placements, ready for final marking and a couple of exams or vivas, which would give us the much-anticipated postgraduate diploma in dietetics that we needed to gain our registration to practice; easy! What I hadn't appreciated — and only discovered when I arrived in Bristol — was that I wouldn't be completing all of my 32 weeks in the city. Instead, I was told that I would have to travel north to Walsall, in the West Midlands, for my 4-week complimentary placement, before immediately moving south to Plymouth for 6 weeks of renal and catering management experience. My National Express student discount card and brand-new suitcases would be well used in the months to come.

The summer of 1985 had seen large-scale public protests and rioting in many cities across England and the St Pauls area of Bristol didn't escape. I arrived at Temple Meads station one Saturday, at the end of the summer, following an epic 19-hour train journey from the north of Scotland. I had my two heavy cases and a rucksack on my back with everything I hoped I would need to see me through the placement. I had no idea where I was going but passed the address I'd been sent to the taxi driver and set off to my new temporary home. The nurses' residence was a 3-storey building at the back of Bristol Royal Infirmary and I had a basic but comfortable cell-like room on the second floor. There was a single bed, a wooden chest of drawers, a small desk space with a wardrobe and a sink opposite. No room to swing a cat but at least it was warm and cosy. On arrival, I was met by the accommodation officer who showed me round, all the while impressing on me all of the security precautions, observing that there had been recent sightings of prowlers and opportunistic thieves. We had shared bathrooms at each end of the corridor and a large kitchen area, which became my first exposure to food mysteriously disappearing from communal fridges and infestations of silverfish all over the floor— yuck! At the far end of the corridor were the coin-operated public phone and a shared bathroom/shower for the whole floor.

On day two, I took a walk into the city centre only to be alerted to a bomb threat in the Broadmead shopping centre by local police. It was an unsettling experience but thankfully I never encountered any problems in all my time in the city.

On the Monday, I turned up for my first day at the dietetic office and knew straight away that I was going to enjoy my time there. Mary Ball was the chief dietitian who introduced me to everyone and sorted out my uniform — a white dress with blue trim. She was even shorter than me and had a bright bubbly character and a big curly mass of hair. There were already two other students on placement — Alice and Nia — and junior (basic grade) dietitians, Paula Hunt and Sally Griffiths were friendly and encouraging, keeping me busy during my induction. Our senior dietitian, Helen, had quite a posh accent and a social life that was quite separate from the rest of us at weekends so I never really felt that I got to know her very well. Sarafina worked as one of the attached community dietitians and Mrs Baker was the friendly clinic receptionist, who was a bit of a mother hen figure, keeping us students right, listening to our news/troubles and sharing bits of hospital gossip. Jane McKiernan joined us from Leeds after a few months as the specialist in liver disease, followed not long after by Karen Bachelor, a newly qualified basic grade from the West Midlands. Anyone who has known or worked with me over the years will be surprised to know that I was quite shy back then and wasn't great at small talk with strangers.

To make things more awkward, I also struggled quite a lot with the West Country accent and found it strange to be referred to as "my lover" by locals. My own accent and Doric dialect also confounded some of the patients I came across on the wards. On one occasion, I approached an elderly man sat up in bed and introduced myself as the student dietitian. To break the ice initially, I asked him if he was fine. I had to repeat myself three times before another patient informed him that I was only asking how he was. To make matters worse, I started taking a diet history from him and couldn't understand what he was saying. Even when I did make it out, I sometimes wasn't familiar with the foods he was eating — faggots, for instance, had never featured on any menu I had ever encountered, not even in the infamous family cooking sessions during first year in Aberdeen!

Over the years working as a dietitian in so many different parts of the country, I have made it a priority to find out early on about any local dishes and the regional terminology for popular items such as bread rolls, pastry goods and fizzy drinks. For example, I was brought up referring to fizzy drinks as "brew", while Lesley and other Glaswegian students had called lemonade "ginger" and students from Yorkshire generally called it "pop." If I was going to be an effective practitioner, I would have to keep a checklist on me so that I could remember to use the local terminology or I'd struggle to estimate peoples' nutritional intake — one of the core competencies of any dietitian. There was also a language of abbreviations and code words that weren't always apparent to the uninitiated. For instance, there was one time when I was working alongside Mary at a small community hospital for the day. She asked me to follow up the case of a patient in one ward while she went to review a couple of patients on the other one. It was the first time I'd been there and a busy nurse had muttered quietly that the lady I was looking for had gone to "Rose Cottage". As she walked away, I realised that I'd have to try and find it myself and spent half an hour walking round the various scattered pre-fab buildings on the hospital site looking at signposts. As I stood outside looking very lost, a porter took pity on me. He smiled knowingly and gently explained that there was no such place: Rose Cottage was ward code and meant that the patient had died. Staff used this term to avoid using the "d" word openly in case it upset any other patients!

Ward notes were also a bit of a minefield and even if you could read the doctors' handwriting, there was then the challenge of understanding abbreviations — often nothing to do with a clinical condition. ESN (educationally sub-normal) is a very subjective, insulting term that thankfully is no longer used to describe a person whose IQ wasn't very high. Another was PITN (pain in the neck). I'm sure that older readers can think of many similar examples. Even today, the same abbreviations can mean different things in different specialities, so staff and students need to be careful not to misunderstand them.

Meanwhile, back at Bristol Royal Infirmary, two new students, Sue and Rachel, had arrived and we all got on well, supporting each other as well as sharing all our daily experiences. Our social life was also great and we were regularly joined by dietitians Jane and Karen on trips to the Arnol Fini cinema, local restaurants and clubs. The variety of places to eat was huge and there was food on offer from so many countries that I thoroughly enjoyed exploring many of them and trying out new things. My lack of experience with lots of menu options did cause a few surprises of course and I recall ordering whitebait in one restaurant, only to have a large bowl of whole, deep-fried fish to crunch my way through, causing great entertainment for everyone. We were kept very fit walking for miles around the corridors and the bowels of Bristol Royal Infirmary, while also navigating our way up all the hills around the city.

It was a time before any prescribed nutritional supplements so the diet cooks made them up in the underground kitchen, using varying concoctions of milk or fruit juice, cream, protein or calorie powders and raw eggs. They were mixed up and portioned into wax cartons which were distributed to the wards on top of the meal trolleys, arriving "nice" and warm... I can't say that they looked appetising or that anyone really enjoyed them, and there was certainly a lot of waste. The same is true today, which is why we have now moved back to a food-first model of nutritional care, enjoyed far better by people who need building up whether they're in hospitals or care homes. It was a memorable happy time and grounded me in so many essential aspects of clinical dietetics that have stuck with me throughout my career. It would encourage me later, as I worked in other parts of the country, to support students to have a good experience in whichever department I was working in. Years later, on my return to Scotland, I was even invited back to RGU to share my experiences and insights with students of the day — a very proud moment.

When the time came to move to Walsall in the autumn, I was reluctant to go as I had grown so much in confidence and made such good friends. I packed my trusty suitcases and rucksack then headed up the motorway network on yet another National Express coach hoping that it would be a good experience. It was going to be a much smaller dietetic department than I was used to but the work was very complimentary to Bristol, where I had learned so much about Afro-Caribbean foods. The West Midlands has a high

Asian population and I loved exploring all the small, local shops taking in all the smells and sights of so many things I'd never seen before. I recall one day helping a colleague to set out a colourful array of spices in a variety of presentations ready for someone from medical illustration to photograph them for a set of slides. I had never seen, never mind smelled, so many exotic scents and learned so much about Asian cookery as I did during that time.

It seemed a far cry from catering classes at RGU and my limited knowledge of herbs for cooking! Exploring local shops and markets, I came across a whole new range of foodstuffs, spices, pulses and languages. It would also give me my first experience of working through interpreters, which helped me as I moved to new jobs around the country in later years. The start of my placement at The Manor hospital would have been made much less stressful had mobile phones been invented at the time. I had been asked to meet Joan, the dietetics manager, at a separate small community hospital near the nurses' home where I was to live for 4 weeks. I got there in plenty of time and waited patiently outside the main reception area in the cool September morning air. It would have been easier if each of us had been wearing name badges or if someone on the reception desk had known who either of us were. After three quarters of an hour of searching, Joan had lost patience waiting for me inside the building and nearly knocked me over in her rush to get outside, which helped us introduce ourselves. We managed to laugh the situation off and headed along to the main hospital to meet everyone else in the dietetic department. Joan had worked at the same place for several decades and had a good relationship with all her staff. It transpired that she was a committed vegetarian and one evening, she invited us all to her home for tea. She lived alone with no television and I was impressed to find that she was cultivating a crop of edible mushrooms in a darkened spare room. So much of how she lived amazed me and I soon learned how good vegetarian food could be. She prepared a wonderful spicy, stuffed marrow and lentil dish for us all, which went down a treat as I hadn't been eating as well as usual. I found Walsall quite a lonely place, especially as the nights grew darker. Living in the staff residences, I rarely saw anyone else and the TV lounge was always empty but I managed to keep in touch with news from home by way of a weekly phone call from the public call box downstairs. I made the most of the situation by listening to lots of music. I had several pre-recorded cassette tapes that I took everywhere with me on my travels, and I also had my trusty portable radio. Whenever I hear the Waterboys song 'Whole of the Moon', it takes me straight back to my time there.

All dietitians need to be able to teach individuals in small or large groups using a range of learning styles or formats. It's important that we communicate in a way that supports people to understand the theory and practicalities of how nutrition can improve their health whatever condition they happen to be living with. Student dietitians were usually allocated a variety of talks to prepare and deliver, under the supervision of a qualified colleague who would mark our teaching plans, knowledge and presentation style. I was fortunate, with hindsight, to get lots of this experience with a wide range of patient groups; far more, in fact, than any of my classmates from Aberdeen. You had a choice of using either a slide projector, complete with a carousel, or an overhead version, which projected whatever you had written onto acetate sheets placed on top of it. The overhead projectors (OHPs) were large, unwieldy machines that I struggled to lift and position correctly. Many departments didn't even have their own one and had to book them out of the Medical Illustration Department for talks. The development of portable OHPs transformed our ability to deliver training in different settings outside the hospital, but it would take many years before they were routinely available.

Both had their challenges: you had to know how to input photographic slides — upside down and back to front — so that they could be properly viewed. Meanwhile, the acetate pens used to draw the images were very pungent and could make you feel quite woozy and lightheaded if you didn't use them in a well-aired room. The water soluble ones weren't so bad but they smudged easily and we soon learned to make sure that we didn't accidentally get them wet or rub them against our clothes — so many hard lessons learned from harsh experience!

On one such occasion in Walsall, I was asked to give a talk to an evening antenatal class. I prepared well and had quite a few prompt cards to remind me of the key messages I had to get across. When we arrived at the hall, there was a far bigger crowd of people than I had ever spoken to before but I was so reassured by the cards in my pocket, that I thought I could get through it okay. The lead midwife introduced me to the group, switched the main hall light off and left the room. As I started to speak, I realised with horror that it was now too dark to see my handwritten notes and I would have to be prompted instead by the slides as they moved forward. I somehow stumbled through the talk but I think I have probably erased everything about that session from my mind in an act of self-preservation; it must have also been quite uncomfortable for the expectant crowd to endure... I left the hall that evening relieved to have finished it and happy knowing that I had a few days off.

I headed out to catch yet another National Express coach, from Digbeth bus station in Birmingham, all set to travel back to Aberdeen for my graduation ceremony two days later. I was looking forward to being there and the prospect of catching up with my family and university classmates. Unfortunately, the journey was not as straightforward as I might have hoped and came to have strong parallels with the film 'Planes, Trains and Automobiles'. I sat waiting in the bus station daydreaming and got quite a shock as I noticed that the Aberdeen coach had started to leave. A sympathetic bus driver took pity on me standing in front of him, close to tears, weighed down by my rucksack and case. He explained that the coach drivers all stopped in the same motorway service station going north and if I got on his coach, he would "hopefully" get me swapped onto the right one. So, sometime later, in the dead of night, I was successfully transferred onto another one bound for Dundee, where I would then "hopefully" be able to re-join my original coach. Miraculously, that's exactly what happened and I arrived in Aberdeen on time, completely exhausted but happy to have made it for the big day with everyone at The Beach Ballroom.

I walked all the way up to Union Street to get my well-worn court shoes re-heeled and I bought a container of navy shoe colouring to make sure they were smartened up for the ceremony. On the day, I headed into town to pick up my rented gown and cap before walking to the photographer's studio for the essential graduation photos. About half a mile away, the rain started — not so unusual for Aberdeen in November — and I arrived ready for the photo shoot looking like the proverbial drowned rat! Thankfully, the receptionist took pity on me, helping me to get dried off and presentable enough for a few memorable photos. The afternoon at the Beach Ballroom was full of buzz and excitement with hundreds of students reunited for the first time in months. Lots of my family had made the journey to Aberdeen and there was lots of laughter afterwards as everyone had their photos taken wearing the graduation gown. It was a proud moment to be the first member of my mother's family to graduate from University.

Back in Walsall the next weekend, I was delighted to be visited by Karen, the bubbly basic-grade dietitian from the Bristol team, who was visiting her family for the weekend. We were joined by her boyfriend and went out for a meal, sharing all the news from the Royal Infirmary and The Manor hospital.

I managed to complete my final week of the complimentary placement without any memorable problems and prepared for my next placement down south. We had a disastrous start to the journey though, as the coach driver nearly caused a major emergency when he turned northbound onto the southbound exit at junction 10 of the M6. He had to brake very suddenly with loud warning blasts of horns coming from worried drivers all around us! I always think of that when I'm driving past that junction and remember the lucky escape we all had. I made it safely back to Bristol, stopping over in my old room for one night, before my next coach trip all the way down to Plymouth.

I arrived quite late one cold winter's night in November 1985, and after collecting my keys from the Derriford Hospital reception, I was directed up a dark hill to the staff accommodation block. Dragging my trusty suitcase, I was delighted to see how modern and comfortable the building was compared to what I'd been used to in both Bristol and Walsall. I discovered that I was sharing a lovely five-bedroom flat with a hospital pharmacist called Kevin, an operation dept. assistant called Matt and two others who we rarely saw. On my first day, I was pleased to meet my supervisor, senior renal dietitian, Sharon, who had arranged a busy, varied fortnight of specialist experiences for me. I wasn't expected to give dietetic advice to anyone but I was given lots of opportunity to meet and chat to a wide range of clinical staff and to meet people living with a variety of kidney diseases — some spending life on dialysis — and their families. I saw home haemodialysis in action one day when carrying out domiciliary visits around North Devon with the specialist renal nurse and was amazed to see how well they were coping. It was only with the help of dedicated family members that they were able to manage that way, as they connected themselves to the machines for several hours of treatment three times a week. At least they didn't have to endure long, stressful journeys up to Plymouth but their lives were really challenging and very tiring. The two weeks spent with the renal team left me with a strong sense of the crucial, life-saving role that the complex renal diet has in keeping people safe and well. It is one of the few diets that can cause very serious complications and can easily kill if not explained or followed correctly. The experience stayed with me for years and I often reflected on it when I went on to work as part of a large, regional renal unit in the East Midlands later in my career.

My four weeks of catering management experience was designed to help me appreciate the challenges of implementing large-scale menu-planning and cooking to try and suit the many varied tastes of patients and staff being served throughout the hospital. At one point, Richard, the manager, asked me to carry out a lunchtime waste management project to help his staff understand and compare levels of plate waste across several hospital wards. As you might imagine, this involved a degree of delving through platefuls of wasted or uneaten food and weighing how much patients were leaving on their plates. Never have a pair of blue plastic gloves been more welcome! The smell was awful and, not surprisingly, I've never felt the need to carry out — or ask anyone else to carry out — an audit of plate waste ever again.

The week before Christmas 1985, I left Plymouth with many great memories and lots of useful experience. Little did I know that many years later, I would find myself working in The Highlands alongside Sharon's niece, Charlotte, who has followed her aunt's career path, specialising in diabetes rather than renal disease. UK dietetics is indeed a VERY small profession...

Back in Bristol in January 1986, we had a new," famous" chief dietitian in the form of Pat Howard, who had transferred to work with us from a large teaching hospital in London. She was very highly respected and well known to many in the profession and played a big part in the creation and success of the PENG (parenteral and enteral nutrition group). I took inspiration from her work and hoped to be able to have that same impact and influence as her in my own career.

In the meantime, I continued with a few weeks of supervised ward work before being expected to manage my own in-patient and clinic caseload. The hospital had a number of highly specialist areas of clinical work, including a large, regional liver unit dominated by a revolving door of patients suffering recurrent complications of severe and uncontrolled alcoholism. I saw many very yellow, brightly jaundiced people with huge abdominal ascites, which had to be tapped and drained of fluid. Many of them also had the classic signs and symptoms of spider naevi and bleeding oesophageal varices, causing anaemia, nausea and fatigue. It was a sad place in many respects as lots of patients were repeatedly admitted to the ward and were well known to the specialist clinical staff.

General ward work in Bristol was very varied, which was great because, as a student, you were always looking to be able to tick off new diet treatments that you had explained to patients. The one I always dreaded was the high fibre diet referral. Invariably, the patient was elderly and hard of hearing, situated halfway down a long Nightingale ward. Trying to have a conversation about someone's bowel habits whilst having to constantly repeat what I was saying was cringe-worthy, knowing that surrounding patients and staff were looking on with expressions of pitying bemusement. Nowadays, most students never receive referrals for high fibre diets as written information is often posted out to patients or they may be signposted to them via a web link. The focus in acute wards has now become far more targeted to treating the sickest of people, requiring nutritional support and more complex tube feeding or intravenous (IV) nutrition.

One week, I was assigned some time to shadow nursing staff on the specialist eating disorders unit, which treated people with anorexia alongside those who were morbidly obese and awaiting major surgical weight loss interventions such as jejunal bypass and jaw wiring. It was my first exposure of bariatric interventions and I observed that there were no specialist scales. Instead, patients had to be taken down to the kitchen area, where people had to sit on the extra-large potato weighing scales. They were the only ones that could accommodate people who were heavier than 25 stones. It was quite an embarrassing and undignified situation for all concerned. Back on the wards, there were even occasions when two beds had to be joined together for some of the much larger patients. Today, there is routine access to bariatric furniture, equipment and facilities so that patients no longer have to go to the kitchen area to be weighed. I was shocked to learn that when others were having their jaws wired up, some patients had to have a tooth removed at the front of their mouth, allowing them to insert a straw to suck up a liquid diet. They were also supplied with a pair of wire cutters in case they started to choke and needed to release their jaws quickly to allow any vomit or aspirate to be coughed up. Some of the more determined patients found their past temptations too much, though, and would even liquidise chocolate bars and mousses.

Very restrictive new 600kcal liquid diets were also being trialled by Paula and the specialist consultant in the bariatric clinic. They had very mixed success, however, as patients struggled to comply with the poor taste, lack of daily variety and constant hunger pains. The introduction of some fat-binding drugs later on had equally poor outcomes as patients experienced embarrassing diarrhoea-type accidents, having succumbed to the temptation of foods that were too high in fat. It didn't matter how many times they were warned about the side effects, many would still see just how far they could push their luck without a sudden explosion of fatty stools rapidly leaving their bowel.

On the gastroenterology unit, a variety of intestinal conditions were diagnosed, treated, and occasionally, required surgery. I saw lots of examples of people struggling to live with Crohn's disease and inflammatory bowel disease. They were often starved to empty their bowel, allowing it to rest before having to introduce very specialist elemental feeds. They smelled and tasted revolting and often had to be given with a cup which had a covered lid. The complex tube feeds that we use commonly today had not been invented so occasionally, the elemental feed would have to be syringed via a nasogastric tube, which could cause virulent diarrhoea, as they were so concentrated. I was invited to spend one morning in clinic with quite a famous consultant gastroenterologist/author of the time and a proactive proponent of the high fibre diet. Patients arrived for internal bowel examinations, having followed strict dietary guidelines designed to empty the colon and rectum, thereby allowing him to get a clear view of any abnormalities or disease. Towards the end of the clinic, I left the room having witnessed several rigid sigmoidoscopies and listened to a variety of conversations about food allergies and irritable bowel habits. I had my own clinic to prepare for that afternoon, which included people with coeliac disease and those who were following very restrictive exclusion diets, gradually re-introducing new foods to their daily meals. I discovered during my clinic that the last lady of the morning session had sadly not followed the rigorous preparation diet and consequently did not cope at all well with the sigmoidoscopy, resulting in a very messy clinic room (the term "explosive" describes it best) and a quickly abandoned appointment. Naturally, the consultant left the nursing team to tidy up while he took an early lunch. A lucky escape for me too... In fact, I've never much fancied specialising in gastroenterology since.

Later, in diabetic clinic, I was shocked to notice that one gentleman had somehow managed to lose about a stone in weight since a recent hospital stay. As many readers will know, one of the common complications of poor diabetic control is neuropathy in the feet, which can often lead to gangrene, resulting invariably to varying degrees of surgical excision. Yes, you've guessed it, the man hadn't lost weight conventionally; he had in fact had a leg amputated! I wasn't the first and I'm sure that I won't be the last student to make that mistake but at least I realised before writing up my clinic notes and reporting back to my supervisor. It created a lot of laughter with the clinic nurses who all thought it was such a silly mistake, having seen it all before.

Early on in 1986, pressure was mounting on me to find somewhere to complete my eleven-week "industrial" placement once my time at the Royal Infirmary had finished. As luck would have it, I was attending a meeting with some dietetic staff from another unit and found myself in conversation with Sue Stocker, a senior dietitian in the Bristol health promotion team, which was based in another part of the city.

It was quickly agreed with RGU that I could stay on in Bristol and carry out my final three months with Sue as my supervisor. I was delighted because it meant that I was able to remain in my room in the nurses' home and keep in contact with the dietetic staff and students from BRI. I went on to successfully complete my 32-week timetable at Bristol Royal Infirmary and seamlessly transferred to work with Sue and the health promotion department. It was a great complimentary experience with lots of exposure to other practitioners specialising in smoking cessation, oral health and weight management. I was given a variety of small projects to carry out and helped at various health fayres, school talks and in leaflet design. The team made my experience really enjoyable and Sue was such a positive person, always smiling and optimistic. She even encouraged me with my first job applications as we looked together at her BDA monthly jobs flier, which was the main way vacancies were advertised across England in those days. Most Scottish posts were advertised in a national newspaper north of the border and invariably tended to go to students who were on placement in local departments. During the spring of 1986, I spotted an advert for maternity leave cover in Yorkshire — at Jimmy's hospital in Leeds — and talked it through with Sue before completing and posting off my application. She was so nice and even invited me to stay for the weekend at her home, over the border in Wales, knowing that I was so far away from home. I was sorry when I eventually had to leave both the health promotion and wider dietetic team, but soon after, I headed off on the coach once again, back to Aberdeen for one final all-day journey. In the years that followed, I bumped into Sue several times at BDA student training events and she continued to be a great encouragement to so many dietetic staff and students over the years. She emailed as she was about to retire, to tell me that she'd followed my career over more than 30 years and wanted to congratulate me on a recent article I had written in "Dietetics Today". Our profession needs more encouraging people like this to guide and support us, especially when life can be challenging.

Back at RGU, it was a more relaxed, informal time in classes and tutorials, now only based at the west end Kepplestone campus. We were now the most senior students and no longer in classes 5 days a week. It was the 50th "Golden" anniversary year of the BDA and we were all presented with a commemorative mug in the Association blue and gold colours of the day. One of the final projects we were assigned involved researching a famous name in the field of nutrition and dietetics and presenting their work to the rest of the year and a handful of lecturers. I was given the name Professor Philip James and was aware that he had led the development of the NACNE (National Advisory Committee on Nutrition Education) dietary guidelines at the time, advising the government on promoting a healthier diet for the UK population. I had a moment of inspiration when I realised that he was working as the leading researcher at the Rowett research institute on the outskirts of Aberdeen. I pragmatically decided to save myself some time from studying his work in the library by interviewing him face to face. I made the call to arrange a personal appointment with him, which was accepted, and I headed off on the bus to meet him in his office. He was very genial and humoured me with a two-hour interview, which included lots of personal life stories as well as the work he was famed for. When I presented my findings back at RGU, some of the lecturers were quite horrified to hear that I'd actually dared to go and speak with the great man and I believe that someone even called him to apologise that a student had gone to interview him in person.

When it came to presenting our projects to class-mates and lecturers, I distinctly remember starting off my talk about him by saying: "From a small house in South Wales..." Dr Wise was sat shaking his head despairingly and said afterwards that my presentation sounded more like a story from a woman's weekly magazine! It was hardly the detailed analysis of the hundreds of research papers and topics that they were expecting. His horror was met with muffled sniggers from the rows of students, but I still passed the task... for initiative and effort if nothing else, no doubt. In

June 1986, I finally prepared to leave Robert Gordon's, delighted to have successfully completed my post graduate diploma in Dietetics. There was no option in Scottish Universities to carry out a further Masters or PhD at that time, so I quickly posted the handwritten paperwork needed to register with the CPSM (Council for Professions Supplementary to Medicine) as a fully qualified state registered dietitian. At the time, three Scottish universities produced a disproportionately higher number of qualified dietitians than any of the other home countries and, throughout my working life, I was met with a common comment: How come all you dietitians are Scottish?! Well, it seems that shortbread and Scotch weren't the only exports worth having….

Chapter 3 — The early years

Not long afterwards, I was pleased to receive a letter from the personnel team at St James's university hospital in Leeds, inviting me for an interview. After a very early start and a long train journey from Aberdeen, I arrived to discover that there were four locum posts available, with contracts lasting at least six months, which was the maximum time for paid maternity leave back then. We weren't told the outcome on the day and I had to wait once again for the postman to break my suspense. When it came, I had to ring the department from a public call box in Aberdeen and was delighted to be offered my first job, starting on the 6th of July 1986, alongside the three other locums — Liz, Leigh and Alison. My state registration confirmation still hadn't come through, which meant that I couldn't actually start to practice alone and unsupervised. Instead, my first week was

used for induction and shadowing qualified staff —
Sue, Claire and Linda — familiarising myself with diet
sheets, paperwork and the vast maze of corridors,
wards and clinics around the huge hospital site. I
had some temporary, basic accommodation in the
upper floor of the main hospital building but soon
met another new starter — a physio called Linda —
and we made plans to try and find a flat together
as soon as possible. The dietetic department was a
large, busy team, headed up temporarily by Carol
Middleton, while Margaret, the permanent head of
dietetics, was on maternity leave. Carol was a very
experienced renal dietitian who eventually went on
to receive an OBE for her contribution to sports nutrition about ten years later. Our paths have crossed
many times over the years, usually linked to a BDA
committee or conference, and most recently at the
2018 European Federation of Dietetic Associations'
event in Rotterdam, where I was presenting some
award-winning work from The Highlands on nutrition prescribing. Another key figure from Leeds was
the chief paediatric dietitian, Anita MacDonald, now

world-famous Prof MacDonald OBE, managing the dietetic team and leading the way at Birmingham Children's Hospital. She was, and continues to be, a very inspiring professional and it seemed she was able to produce a never-ending series of research and audit reports. Her work ethic was legendary and she spent many more unpaid hours on the wards than she was contracted for. The ward rotations were very varied and gave us basic grades a great mixture of clinical practice with both in-patients and clinics.

The general office, shared by six of us and any students on placement, was on the ground floor of the hospital, with windows facing out, looking onto the business of passers-by in the hospital grounds. It was a huge room with a high ceiling and a large, imposing wooden door, which had to be locked behind you when going off to our wards or to the nearby toilets. There was a large planter in one corner, near the kettle, containing a less-than-healthy-looking yucca. It might have stood more of a chance had staff not taken to pouring dregs from their old coffee mugs into the soil, rather than walking down the corridor to wash them out in the bathrooms, but that would have meant locking and unlocking the big door; too much hassle for most.

One morning, we returned to the office to find Sue, one of the senior dietitians, deep in calculations and textbooks. Thinking she must have a very complex case to research, we sat quietly writing up our notes. Eventually, someone asked her why she was looking so puzzled, and it transpired that the patient was rather different to the ones we were dealing with. She was trying to work out a diet plan for a senior registrar's pet gerbil that had been off colour! Needless to say, she didn't get very far with that and was soon called back to the reality of ward visits.

Outside of work, I was soon sharing a house in the Harehills area of town with three physiotherapists — Mary, Cheryl and Linda — who I'd met upstairs in our hospital accommodation; life was never dull. We often saw each other around the hospital but never had to work directly together.

On one occasion on the ward, I was asked to speak with a French tourist who'd been admitted and needed help organising a diabetic diet for him from the kitchen. I thought I'd put my sixth year language skills to the test and attempted to take a diet history from him in French. Other patients on the ward listened with curious amusement while the man himself appeared to find it quite bewildering... We soon re-started when he asked me — very fluently — if it might be easier for us to talk in English! Down in the diet kitchen, I relayed the story to Beryl, our catering assistant, who clucked around us all like a mother hen, occasionally tut-tut-ting if we were late notifying her about new diets or products that needed ordering. At that time, dietitians were also expected to go to the catering office each day to check and code patients' weight-reducing and diabetic menu choices, noting the number of scoops of potato that they were allowed at each meal and ensuring that they only had "healthy" choices. A scoop of mash equated to 10g of carbohydrate and people trying to lose weight were often only able to have one at a meal. There were rarely other options of starchy carbohydrate available at mealtimes. In those days, we even had to come in at weekends to do it and were expected to be available for an on-call rota over bank holidays in case there were any urgent dietetic queries or unexpected therapeutic diets that needed organising. I had to carry out two days of on-call cover during the Christmas holidays of 1986, having just returned from a week's holiday in The Gambia. I arrived back to my frost-covered house, which was so cold that I could hardly get the front door to shut behind me. I slept in front of the gas fire in the kitchen, with my notes and textbooks nearby, to be warm and near to the landline just in case a call came through from Jimmy's switchboard. Thankfully, I didn't have any calls and was able to head back to the North of Scotland to see my family soon after. Through a mixture of circumstances, I was fortunate in being able to stay working with the Jimmy's dietetic team until February 1987 and enjoyed getting to grips with the challenges of the maxillo-facial unit, which involved lots of tube-feeding regimens. The options available were fairly rudimentary and still fairly limited in variety. It was years before we had Schofield equations or PENG handbooks to calculate individuals' nutritional requirements. It was really gritty stuff and quite a traumatic time for the patients undergoing pioneering, really gruelling treatment. They often had cancerous growths on their tongues, or inside their mouths or jaws, which could appear quite frightening and had an awful smell. It was important not to let them see how shocked you might be seeing them and smelling the odour around them. They really appreciated being treated as though nothing was out of the ordinary and it helped them relax at the prospect of what was to come in intensive care, after surgery. It was truly a great team effort to support patients and their families through life-changing, frightening times, developing what is now a well-advanced mainstream form of treatment for people with head and neck cancers.

I tried applying for lots of jobs during January and February 1987 and had no problem getting interviews. Frustratingly at that time, there were far more newly qualified dietitians than vacancies and I struggled to get past that initial stage. I always seemed to be just pipped at the post and spent several uncertain weeks in the ranks of the unemployed until, out of the blue one day, I was finally offered another fixed-term contract; this time it was in Sheffield. The dietetic manager, Susan Jones, had interviewed me previously and decided to invite me to work with the team at The Royal Hallamshire Hospital in the city's west end. Every day, I took the train and bus from my home in Leeds, pleased to have the chance to get some more dietetic experience and to progress my career. It was only a three-month opportunity but offered a good variety of clinical work alongside a happy team of staff, always positive and encouraging each other. Out-patient clinics brought a wide mix of people needing advice about a good range of specialist diets. Taking diet histories could often be quite amusing and I can remember several patients over the years who were adamant that they had *semi-skilled* milk in their tea. I have lost count of the times people told me that they "hardly eat anything" only to uncover just how many packets of crisps, biscuits, alcoholic drinks and takeaways, etc., they were actually having "just once or twice a week"! One elderly gent came for help and advice about his high fibre diet, explaining that he wasn't having much success using the laxatives and didn't think much of the suppositories that the GP had prescribed for him to use. He explained that the pain of inserting them was too much because the foil was scratching his bottom so badly that it was sometimes bleeding! Weighing and measuring peoples' height meant asking them to take off their heavy coats, shoes or boots... we kept a can of air freshener in the desk drawer, which was essential for many windowless clinic rooms, especially in the height of summer when sweaty feet, sticking to the scales, were the norm! Measuring someone's height also meant getting up close to people as we reached above them to bring the measuring stick down on their heads. I had to develop the skill of quickly checking the height of many very odorous patients, while holding my breath and simultaneously talking to them. If they had bad breath as well, it was extra challenging, and we might excuse ourselves to step outside while they put their shoes back on.

We were part of a really positive, diverse network of dietitians from all the other Sheffield hospitals-

Weston Park, The children's hospital, The Royal Hallamshire and the mental health unit. We organised joint in-service training days and met up with many other colleagues across the county at BDA Yorkshire branch meetings. It's good to see that it continues to thrive and receive recognition at BDA awards ceremonies over the years. The commitment of dietitians, willing to share and network, has remained very popular and it is well attended and a good source of CPD (Continued Professional Development) for many dietitians in the area.

My locum post came to an end in May 2007 and I faced the prospect of unemployment once again. Susan suggested that I apply for a senior post across the city at The Northern General Hospital. I knew many of the staff because of the good network that we already had and I was delighted to be selected for interview. The manager, Sue, and her deputy, Val Jacob, interviewed me, and, despite feeling very pressured, I was offered my first permanent job; the relief was overwhelming. In the period between the two jobs, I kept myself occupied with dietetic-related activities and I successfully applied as a volunteer for a place working on a children's diabetes camp, which The British Diabetic Association (now Diabetes UK) ran annually. It was generally considered to be a desirable addition to any junior dietitian's curriculum vitae.

Fortunately, I was selected to work for a week in July, as part of a dietetic team in one camp, at an outdoor centre near Tavistock in Devon. Gill Welsh was the lead dietitian for the week, and we worked together with two others to develop varied menus, preparing lots of sugar-free squash, snacks, meals and packed lunches for the children who were all aged 10-12. I remember the first morning they came down for breakfast and we noticed a very distinct smell of mint in the air. On closer inspection, we realised that it was coming from the boys, who had 'gelled' their hair with clear mint toothpaste! It was the first time away from home for many of them and they kept us on our toes, trying to keep up with all their activities and antics. On a positive personal note, I managed to successfully kick my habit of taking two sugars in my coffee: there just wasn't any available so I just got used to not having it.

In August 1987, on return from the diabetes camp, I started my new permanent job with the team at The Northern General Hospital, working as a specialist senior 1 (band 7) dietitian in the regional burns and plastic surgery unit. Other team members at the time included basic grades Anne Daly, Jackie Wilkinson and Lynn Harbottle. Senior staff included Val Naylor, Fiona Ford and Liz Jolly — our very posh-spoken mental health specialist, who travelled around the various hospital sites in Sheffield, complete with her Harrods shopping bag, using public transport. Our secretary at the time was Linda, a larger-than-life, breezy Yorkshire mum, who kept the department running smoothly. She managed all the office appointments and the workloads of dietitians who relied on her to type letters, etcetera. Like many staff in her role, she was something of an agony aunt, who patiently listened to all our woes — whether work or romantic — and knew all the hospital gossip. She was a very clever lady in her own right, of course, and aspired to greater things, so she also studied for an English degree in her spare time. I was often reminded of the title character in

'Educating Rita' when listening to her experiences of being a mature student, juggling motherhood, work and her degree. One day, she arrived at work clearly very upset because the previous night, she had spent hours writing a long essay on her computer, only for her husband to come along and unplug it to use the power socket for something else he wanted to do. She lost all of her evening's work and had to take herself off to a hot bubble bath with a large glass of red stuff to try and calm down. Needless to say, she managed to finally get her essay finished and continued with her studies, passing with flying colours.

The Northern General Hospital in Sheffield is spread over a very large site, and, at the time I was in post, there were two quite different parts to it, having had additional buildings added over the years. Our offices were situated in an old out-patient building near the entrance to the main hospital site, which meant that we all had to be very organised to avoid having to spend lots of time walking backwards and forward to ward areas — especially when the weather was bad! At one time or another, we all experienced the discomfort and inconvenience of being caught in heavy showers — steam rising from us as we sat drying off by a radiator back in the office — or slipping and sliding in the snow or ice of the challenging Sheffield winters. Good preparation was essential, so I always made sure that my folder of diet sheets and forms contained enough to cover all eventualities for the morning or afternoon ahead. The pockets of my standard-issue white coat bulged with the requisite notebooks, calculator, pens and nasogastric tubes (in case I had to show one to any patients or relatives). I knew that I would be able to get a coffee and biscuit from a ward kitchen if I needed refreshments during my patient visits but I also took some cash to pick up something for lunch on the way back to the office.

The dietetic service for the health authority was led at the time by Valerie Beattie, a fellow Scot from Aberdeen. She was very dynamic, enthusiastic and positive and certainly a great inspiration for many of us. She introduced me to the potential of perhaps one day volunteering with the BDA, as she was a member of the national Executive Council, serving at the time as the honorary treasurer. It was later that year, in a Sheffield-wide team meeting, that the opportunity presented itself. In 1987, a vacancy for the position of the local BDA industrial Relations (IR) representative was discussed at one of our regular team meetings. The successful candidate would be required to attend Joint Staff Consultative Committee (JSCC) meetings, sharing consultations and feedback between the staff side and management. There would also be reporting and information-sharing with the BDA national networks. Val Naylor, one of the senior dietitians, encouraged me to stand for the role and, before I knew it, I had been elected by the rest of the dietetic team. That was the start of a career-long working relationship, volunteering with the BDA in a variety of roles. It was the days of the three big public sector unions — NUPE, NALGO and COHSE — and a few years before they would go on to merge and form UNISON. I found myself representing the BDA and two other Professions Allied to Medicine (PAM) groups — the physiotherapists (CSP) and OTs (BAOT) — before they started receiving trade union services from UNISON.

I learned so much about the business and politics of the local health service, its key players and all the NHS issues of the day. It shaped my interest in more strategic health politics and I ultimately went on to chair the hospital JSCC myself.

Chapter 4 — Burning challenges.

Working as a burns specialist was often challenging and opened my eyes to the many ways that both adults and children were harmed by steam, heat, lightning and fire. It was full of great experiences with the many benefits of working as an integral, valued member of a close multi-disciplinary team. The burns ward was a "closed unit" to minimise throughput and potential sources of outside infection reaching very vulnerable, compromised patients. It meant that we had to enter via a changing area to don protective gowns and (shared) theatre clogs before coming into contact with anyone inside. Ward rounds were held weekly to ensure that all aspects of care and concern were shared and discussed together. They included: Sandy Miller, a consultant plastic surgeon, Donal, the Irish paediatrician, Pam, the physiother-apist, Sue from OT, Judith, the charge nurse, me from dietetics and occasionally a social worker. Her work was largely, but not exclusively, focused on the children who would appear with potential non-accidental injuries (NAIs) — harmed more often than not by their parents, most commonly by evidence of "dipping" where children had been held in very hot water as a punishment. At one point, an Icelandic microbiologist joined the team to help prevent and treat the risk from open wounds, which are so prone to infections. Karl was travelling around for 3 years with his family, working in several burns centres across Europe, and was an important source of advice about the best way to manage the various strains of bacteria associated with so many open wounds. Our eyes were opened to the dangers of trailing cables on kettles and hot irons, which could easily be pulled down onto toddlers busy exploring their surroundings below. It was the first experience I had of anything like this and I absorbed the way the team dealt with some very challenging conversations.

I can recall several very nasty burn injuries to adults during that time. One was a car mechanic who was lying on his back welding under a car when it caught fire. He suffered 70% burns and remained on the ward for several months, enduring agonising skin grafts, dressing changes and uncomfortable splint positioning of his hands and feet to prevent joint contractures. Another was a young worker who was admitted from the local steel works one day having somehow been caught under a spillage of molten metal. Sadly for him and his family, this was ultimately fatal. On one particularly hot weekend, a fairly new medical consultant was admitted, following an incident at home in his back garden, which happened as a result of him squirting a flammable liquid onto a hot BBQ to light the coals faster. Although his burns weren't deep, they were extremely painful — not to mention embarrassing — requiring a few nights' care and treatment on the ward. I'm sure that he never made that mistake again! I can also recall many of the small children we treated on the unit and the challenges of helping them to receive the nutritional requirements they needed to help them heal and recover successfully. They often needed tube feeds as they were usually put off eating because of their painful burns, dressing changes and the associated upsetting smell from open wounds. The range of specialist paediatric feeds was very limited at that time, which meant that we often had to prescribe other oral nutritional supplements and high calorie snacks between meals to try and improve their chances of making a good recovery. One toddler had been keen to help his dad wash the car one Sunday and somehow managed to knock the bucket of very hot water over himself. Another had pulled a kettle of hot water over his chest and arms but consoled himself by playing with, and talking to, his collection of plastic dinosaurs – even taking them into his bath for the painful dressing changes. One little girl had stood too close to the electric fire, setting fire to her nylon nightie, resulting in full thickness burns over most of her body, which meant that she stayed on the unit for many months. It was agonising to watch them all and I just wished I could do more to help to improve nutritional care, so, I decided to join forces with other colleagues across the UK.

I set about forming the BDA Burns Interest Group, bringing together colleagues from many of the major burns units in England at the time. Nutritional care of burns patients was still in its infancy and there were actually no national, specialist guidelines for clinicians to follow. Many of us used the Sutherland calculations while others adapted the standard national nutrition reference values. The Elia and Schofield equations had yet to be fully developed and adopted but BAPEN (British Association of Parenteral and Enteral Nutrition) have continued to lead the way in standardising more objective nutritional calculations, refining them over the years by building on emerging science and practical experiences. Members of the Burns Interest Group worked collectively to develop the inaugural national dietetic guidelines that were more specific to our patient group and I was really proud to lead on getting these published in 1991. We all had a common purpose and were equally enthusiastic about the potential of our new group. One of the first things we did was to conduct a survey of our units' varying approaches to burns nutrition, which let us compare how practice differed or aligned. It was important to try and create a standardised model of nutritional assessment and care and we all learned so much from the exercise. I had the opportunity of presenting this work in 1989 at a meeting of The British Burns Association (BBA), being held just up the M1 from Sheffield, at a large conference centre near Wakefield. It was well received, and I was completely stunned to be approached afterwards by the chair who offered me the chance to represent British burns dietitians with the BBA contingent at the upcoming conference of international burns associations in Delhi. It also meant participating in a further week-long study tour of India, organised and paid for by the BBA, the Indian Burns Association (IBA) and The British consulate. Naturally, I said yes – what an honour! Not for the last time, I found myself in the right place at the right time. In the autumn of 1990, I met up with the rest of the team at the airport for our trip to India and got chatting with Charmaine, a small bubbly research nurse from Manchester who had just completed her PhD. All the others were medics — plastic surgeons to be precise — and we found out early on that there was a very stark distinction in the way we would be treated as nurses and AHPs, compared to medics.

Landing in Delhi in the late evening, my senses were overwhelmed as I stepped out onto the tarmac — the heat, smells and sights were so different to what I'd left behind in Sheffield. We were escorted to our hotel in a team minibus and, en route from the airport, Charmaine and I discovered that someone had booked the two of us into a local YMCA hostel. This was in stark contrast to the medics who were to stay in the more luxurious surroundings of the Delhi Hilton. Fortunately for us, the medics insisted that we should also stay there and so we were saved from the very basic conditions for which we had been destined. The conference was a great experience and some of the other UK burns dietitians had also been able to fly out to participate. The sessions were full of contrasting presentations, with Middle Eastern countries sharing their research, conducted in state-of-the-art burns units compared with the local Indian teams who were forced, by economic circumstances, to work in far more basic settings with limited resources. We heard of some incredible treatment for burns In Delhi, involving potato skins! Local restaurants were being paid to save their potato peelings and they would be collected for use in the hospitals, once they'd been heated to disinfect them and remove any flesh. Closer investigation revealed that rather than healing being due to the potato skins, the medical teams were applying Flamazine (a specialist cream used on burns) before using the skins as a dressing — not quite the miracle use for potatoes we had thought but a good way of recycling their skins. We were all very shocked to learn that many hospitals were treating injuries caused by honour burns, where women were being deliberately scalded with boiling water or burned in some other way. There were also many accidental burns, caused by clothing catching alight from the sparks and flames of open fires, which many poorer families still relied on for cooking. It was quite a revelation for us to hear some of their stories as we toured around a variety of burns units to see for ourselves. It was also quite levelling to observe firsthand the basic clinical conditions where patients were be cared for, with relatives often sleeping on the floor under their beds and preparing their meals for them. At the conference, I also enjoyed the opportunity to meet so many burns specialists from across the UK, including many senior consultants in other burns units who were all interested to understand more about my role and the importance of good nutritional care. One of them was Michael Masser, a consultant from another Yorkshire burns and plastics unit, at Pinderfields Hospital in Wakefield — more of which later... Towards the end of week one, those of us who would be going on to participate in the study tour of Bombay were treated by the IBA to a trip to the Taj Mahal – and what an experience it was! Walking through the entrance gate, I was completely blown away by the sight of it; well worth the very early start to the day and the long train journey to Agra. I reminded myself that I wouldn't have been able to have this amazing experience if I hadn't co-ordinated a survey of nutritional care in English burns units. I hope that will be an encouragement, to anyone starting out in their career, to make the most of any seemingly insignificant opportunity that comes your way because you never know where it will lead!

Two days after that amazing part of my trip, I found myself en route to our next venue and I still find it amusing to remember that the flight to Bombay on Indian Airways was my first (and only) experience of eating curry for breakfast. To add to the unique encounter, a crew member had passed through the cabin spraying some sort of disinfectant over us before we took off, so the food was then tainted by the remaining odour from whatever residual liquid we had on us and in our nostrils. Once we'd landed and gathered at the exit with our luggage, Charmaine and I were whisked off to our accommodation in a waiting taxi. Thinking that we would be meeting up with the others at the hotel, our hearts sank when we pulled up outside a YMCA building, which was ominously situated on the top floor of a drug rehab clinic. There was no running water or toilet (just a hole in the far corner of the floor), the mattresses on the beds appeared to have patches of horsehair stuffing sticking through them and several ravens were sat squawking menacingly on the rusting iron railings outside. Once the sense of shock had lifted and I was able to think properly, it didn't take long before I decided to involve the British consul, who was part-sponsoring our trip. She was in the middle of a BBQ at home but audibly gasped when I phoned to tell her where we were. She then came straight over to pick us up in her lovely, air-conditioned car, to take us to join the rest of our colleagues who were staying at the 5-star Oberoi hotel. The American team were equally bemused though they were rather unsettled by the way nurses and AHPs were being treated so differently to doctors. The next day, we were even more shocked when our hosts moved the two of us out of the Oberoi to a three-star hotel in another area of Bombay; my room over-looked a local hospital, allowing me to see patients being treated in the wards. We never quite knew what was going to happen to us next, but we were picked up by different people each day and taken to join the others at whichever venue we were due to speak at with everyone else.

In my ignorance of international speaking, I had travelled all the way to India with a full slide carousel in my large suitcase together with a variety of OHP acetates – ready for anything I could think we might have to speak about. The American consultant in our group found this quite quaint! Nowadays, of course, we would simply email our presentations to the organisers or use digital platforms to share our work, eliminating the need to carry a heavy suitcase full of teaching materials. We all delivered teaching sessions at a variety of settings and I was also invited to speak with groups of student dietitians at the local university, which was a great experience that remains with me today, inspiring me to share my work and learning at conferences and settings across the world. The staff were always so welcoming and grateful to us all for our presentations and even prepared some lunch for us, brought in from home in traditional Tiffin dishes. The hospitality of the Indian people was very generous but my delicate Scottish palate wasn't quite prepared for the heat of the spices in many of the foods, so I struggled to eat very much other than the chapatis! One evening, we were treated to an evening out at a plush Bombay country club, which was clearly an exclusive venue for the wealthier people of the city. The IBA team arranged for a grand buffet with a tasty selection of dishes and accompaniments and as they wanted us to feel more at home, they had even prepared their own version of fish and chips!

Throughout our week in Bombay, we had several opportunities to visit local hospitals to see how burns care and health services were delivered in India. It was quite a contrast to the NHS we were used to, which had the positive effect of making us all the more appreciative of our own workplaces. We had some nice downtime too and I was very pleased when our team was joined for coffee one morning by none other than Dr Elsie Sutherland — an expert in the field of burns care — who had developed the unique formula for calculating the nutritional requirements of patients, which many of us used back in the UK. She spent the day with us and joined us for a pre-arranged boat trip across to Monkey Island, a short journey across the water from the hustle and bustle of the city. It was a popular tourist spot and naturally there were lots of traders trying to sell us things, but I was drawn to one stall where an eye-catching array of semi-precious stones was set out to tempt us. I bought a rather grey-looking stone, about 5" across, which split apart to reveal some lovely Amethyst — my birthstone — and it has travelled with me to every house I've lived in for all these years; a tangible reminder of my trip to India. Despite enjoying the whole experience, my fragile Scottish constitution had constantly struggled with the dry Indian heat, noise and business of Indian city life so I was glad to set off home via Bombay airport at the end of the week. It was a surreal experience in many ways as we had to first weigh our own luggage before checking in. Once my trusty suitcase had disap-peared on the conveyer belt, I realised that I still had some family presents in my cabin bag. The check-in assistant hardly batted an eyelid when I pulled out a wooden fish, which opened up to reveal a sharp, cere-monial dagger inside. I thought he would confiscate it but instead he told me to walk airside through a side door where I could look for my own suitcase to stow it away safely! I couldn't imagine that happening at any UK airport but was pleased to quickly find my bag, lying amongst the others on the tarmac, ready to load, and pack my gifts inside. By then, I couldn't wait to finally get onto the air-conditioned plane and was absolutely over the moon to find myself being randomly elevated to business class, which I adapted to very easily; though I have yet to have the experience of "turning left" at an aeroplane door again in all my subsequent travels.

Back to reality of work in Sheffield, I noticed that there was an increasing overlap between my ward work on plastic surgery and the Intensive Care Unit (ITU), when patients had extensive maxillo-facial re-configuration surgery. My previous experience of this in Leeds helped me, of course, and I gradually started working more closely with the local ITU team. I began to receive more referrals for patients needing tube feeds (still a relatively new option), which was a great breakthrough, as they had previously only contacted dietitians once patients were ready to start eating a light diet again, and only then so that we could liaise with the catering department to order them. When a new, purpose-built cardiac intensive care unit was created on site, to include facilities for heart transplants, I was delighted to be released from other general ward work to support patients on both ITUs, along with burns, plastics and the coronary care unit (CCU). The work on my wards was both varied and interesting and I learned so much as part of all the trauma teams. In my head, I had somehow become the glamorous dietitian who had once spoken to my class back in third year at RGU. I even had my own bleep (hospital pager) which was something of a status symbol in those days.

I loved the challenges; the unusual, busy caseload combined with the background stories of the patients' injuries, diagnoses, treatment options and family dynamics. I was used to seeing quite traumatic sights and considered myself pretty unshakable. I coped most of the time by reminding myself that it was the patient who was experiencing the various procedures and treatment rather than me, so I had no excuse for feeling queasy. The one exception to this was finding myself anywhere near the chest physiotherapists when they suctioned patients — even now just thinking about the noise of sputum whirling up the tubes...!

The greatest test of my career came suddenly one Saturday in April 1989, while I was shopping in Liverpool of all places. As I waited in the station lounge for the late train back to Sheffield, reports were coming through on the TV news channel about a serious incident at Hillsborough football ground, home of Sheffield Wednesday. It wasn't until I got home that I understood the horror of what had happened. Today, of course, we can watch events unfold on our mobile phones but back then, we had to wait for news programmes on terrestrial television or radio. I realised that a major incident plan was underway in the local acute hospitals. I called the main ITU to offer my assistance but by then, they had more staff than they could accommodate and were focusing on managing the volume of people coming through the A&E department. I waited and watched helplessly the TV updates (no Twitter, satellite news or mobile phone texts back then), completely stunned at the terrible situation unfolding. By the time I got to work on the Monday, both our ITUs were full and I was kept very busy for the rest of the week, as we supported the survivors from the tragedy. During quiet times in the evening and weekends, there were visits from royalty, senior NHS management and football players. Our team focused more on treating the patients and supporting their loved ones. It was shocking to see some of them pictured on the pages of newspapers and, naturally, very upsetting for many of the families involved. I arrived on the ward one afternoon to a sense that something was about to happen and turned round to see Kenny Dalgleish, Bruce Grobbelaar, Peter Beardsley and a couple of other Liverpool players walking in. They spoke with the anxious relatives and the patients who were able to speak, as many were still unconscious. Their presence was obviously really appreciated by everyone and they made a point of not rushing, taking time to listen while offering comforting words to each. All the clinicians on the ward were lined up and Kenny took the opportunity of offering his thanks for everything we were doing— it was a humbling moment. At a JSCC meeting a couple of weeks later, some staff were clearly still very upset by the whole experience and a couple expressed how guilty they felt that they hadn't been able to help more. It would take many months for things to settle down on the wards again. Our chief executive, Neil McKay (now Lord McKay), handled it all calmly. He was a popular, down-to-earth figure with staff, unions and Trent regional health authority and later went on to work as an advisor at the Department of Health. Before he left Sheffield, I managed to secure him as a speaker at one of the first BDA regional stewards' conferences in Ironbridge, Shropshire. He gave insights and credibility to working alongside management and the importance of working in strong partnership by helping staff to listen and respect each other's concerns and positions on contentious topics, something that we were all able to relate to.

In the following year, there was more tragedy to come as news of a violent incident at neighbouring Pinderfields Hospital reached us on the burns unit. We were all very shocked to hear about the tragic death of Michael Masser, who some of us had met in India. Along with another consultant colleague, he had been murdered in his out-patient clinic by a schizophrenic patient who stabbed them in a fit of rage. Sadly, despite the best, heroic efforts of terrified colleagues, neither of the men could be saved. Michael's death affected all NHS workers who knew and respected him in the field of the burns and plastic surgery. There were many other sad and challenging situations during my formative years at The Northern General but one further case has always stuck in my mind. A young woman with cystic fibrosis was a regular on both ITU and the respiratory ward as her lungs struggled to cope with the complications of the condition. Like so many CF patients, she also struggled to maintain even a low healthy weight and I got to know her and her family quite well as we talked so much about her diet, tested out different flavours of newly emerging nutritional supplements and generally tried to stop her feeling too bored with hospital food. She was a happy, resilient person, even in the dark times, and we were all so happy to hear that she had become engaged to her school sweetheart. Sadly, she passed away not long after that (she was only 24) and I took the decision — along with several ward colleagues who had known her well — to attend her funeral. I have never chosen to do that again because the inconsolable grief of her mother having to be almost dragged out of the funeral car into the crematorium was one of the most upsetting things I have ever witnessed. I realised early in my career that I had become too emotionally involved in the life of a patient and needed to step back within my professional boundaries, while still remaining sympathetic and compassionate. It was an important lesson but one that many NHS staff struggle with at various points in their working life — we are a caring profession after all.

Around the same time, a recently qualified dietitian called Claire Plester joined the Northern General department. She was a very bright, bubbly person with a soft Irish accent who was really enthusiastic about exploring and developing new approaches in nutrition support. We became aware of work being trialled in Northampton by Christine Russell's team, where they had been piloting jejunal feeding, which was pretty ground-breaking back then. Claire persuaded one of our general surgeons to purchase some jejunal feeding packs and they started to pilot inserting and using them with patients during oesophageal surgery instead of using TPN (a very expensive, risky form of intravenous feeding, administered via an arterial neck line). It went very well and more patients soon benefitted from this as the other surgeons became confident about using them routinely for enteral nutritional support. Now, it is such a common approach for artificially feeding people that it's hard to remember a time when we didn't have jejunostomies as an option for nutritional management. It would still be several years before home enteral feeding — never mind home TPN — would liberate people and allow them to care for their own nutritional needs at home, freeing up hospital beds for other patients who were more in need of them. We had a wide mix of regional clinical specialities at the hospital and the dietetic team continued to expand during the four years when I was there. We also took student dietitians on placement from their base at The Royal Hallamshire Hospital, where Susan Jones continued to proactively manage and develop the service.

For a variety of reasons, my manager at The Northern General was completely against having students on placement, but the renal staff and I pressed for a chance to expose them to clinical roles in tertiary care areas for a week or two. I was delighted to become more involved in this because it was a good opportunity for them to see the evolving role of dietetics on the burns and plastic surgery units. I thoroughly enjoyed (and continued to enjoy) working with students and have always been slightly taken aback when I've been approached in meetings or conferences by dietitians who introduce themselves by reminding me that they were once a student of mine and thanking me for inspiring them, which is equally as embarrassing as it is reassuring.

Like most dietetic departments, our lunchtime team meetings often had company representatives attending to tell us about the early, emerging market of oral nutritional supplement (ONS) and associated products. This was a time when ready-made cartons of sip feeds were still being created and there was a lot of competition from companies to persuade us to try and start using new versions, flavours and presentations. One of the first product ranges came from Germany and included flavours like nut, peach and mocha. Other companies created more conventional flavours and it got to the point that we were tripping over products as we had so much choice in our storeroom. We all agreed that it was a far better, more palatable option than making them up from scratch, as had been the norm for many previous years.

It was also always a treat to have reps bringing us a nice lunch of sandwiches, cakes, snacks and juices and there was invariably lots of merchandise too — usually involving versions of stationery items — which we all looked forward to. Our manager also enjoyed the lunches and the free perks, but she had a strong dislike of sales reps, who were doing their best to persuade us to use their products. It got to the point that she would bring in her own alarm clock from home and set a strict time limit of 30 minutes for them to talk, before it rang out loudly! So embarrassing for us all. Over subsequent years, I have worked proactively and respectfully with so many company reps and often saw them move roles to work with competitors and being promoted into more senior, even national roles.

The 1st of August is a day that brings lots of change — and a touch of anxiety — to NHS wards. It's the day that new junior doctors appear, and it can turn the most level-headed professional into a nervous wreck. I always felt sorry for them, as they had to quickly get to grips with all the patients and start to build positive relationships with other staff. For some young staff, that can mean the opportunity for the start of new romantic relationships. One girl was completely focused on finding a man for herself and she became quite obsessional about someone who was working in a neighbouring department. Any opportunity to bump into him, whether in work or on a night out, and the lipstick came out or her hair was quickly re-styled. Fellow colleagues were often roped in to help in her quest. Other staff and students on placement seemed to find her behaviour quite amusing, especially watching as she went into full pursuit mode. With a fresh application of red lipstick and a burst of body spray, she would sweep out of the office as if going into battle. I don't know if she ever got her man, but I've seen the same thing with a variety of colleagues over the years — physios, nurses, managers and others — and some even went on to marry someone they'd met on the wards.

It didn't always go to plan though, and in one case, I recall one lovely girl who was equally determined to "bag" a junior doctor. Once she started going out with one, she was determined to do whatever it took to hold onto him and went a step further by becoming a strict vegetarian to keep him happy. They spent hours commuting between towns on the M1 as she made every effort to see him, even turning up unannounced to cook him surprise meals on his days off. One fateful day, the inevitable happened and she turned up at his hospital flat unexpectedly to find him having an after-noon "lie down" with another woman... Needless to say, the notion of remaining a vegetarian quickly disinte-grated and she headed home via the supermarket where she quickly moved away from her vegetarian life and indulged in her first bacon sandwich in months!

Most afternoons, we took turns to run out-patient clinics and, in some cases, patients could appear from a neighbouring consultant clinic with a referral and sit patiently waiting to be seen. Late one afternoon, I was finishing my paperwork and getting ready to return to the main office when there was a knock on the door. A clinic nurse appeared and asked if I would mind seeing someone new, needing some advice on low cholesterol. I was more than happy to fit him in and waited while she went off to escort him round. A short time later, I heard them approaching outside and as I went to usher him in, I was suddenly stopped in my tracks as I realised that he was actually a very famous public figure, known to many. I suppose I was a bit star-struck and surprised that he would be so down to earth as to attend a general out-patient NHS clinic. Trying not to appear too overwhelmed, I somehow managed to get through a dietetic assessment and offered him some personalised written advice. Sadly, his busy schedule didn't allow him to make a further appointment, so

I never knew whether he took any notice of what I'd suggested, but every time I saw him in newspapers or on TV, I did wonder.

Dietitians in the late eighties, maybe even today, used to dread the clinics in early January and February as they were invariably full of people wanting advice on how to lose weight after overindulging during office parties and family celebrations in November and December. Of course, you will invariably put on more weight when eating and drinking extra treats over the Christmas period, but it would easily come off itself once people got back into their usual daily mealtime routines again. It was never a very fulfilling area of practice for any of us.

One of my colleagues arrived late for work one morning, having missed breakfast, and rushed off round to start her full clinic with a mug of hot tea ready for the first patient of the day. Halfway through listening to a woman talking about her favourite Christmas foods and indulgent treats, she was overcome with hunger and casually pulled a chocolate biscuit from her desk drawer and started eating it as she continued with their consultation. Perhaps unsurprisingly, the patient never did return for a follow-up appointment... Much as that was quite unprofessional, I have never believed that dietitians are the best people to support overweight patients trying to lose weight, except as part of highly specialist bariatric teams, caring for the more morbidly obese group of patients. When you think about it, most dietetic departments are often only able to offer a maximum of four appointments, starting with an initial thirty-minute assessment and then three subsequent fifteen-minute follow-ups over several months. There's no way you can really get to know and support someone well enough in that time to offer any kind of effective treatment. Many people preferred commercial weight management models of group sessions, which are popular for the ongoing encouragement and motivation from others. These days, there are also apps, other digital platforms and self-help options, as well as pre-packaged, calorie-controlled personalised meal deliveries. The causes of obesity are such a complex, multi-facetted physiological, social and psychological challenge and I firmly believe that the public deserve to receive the person-centred support that suits them best with the proviso that it must be based on sound evidence. Nowadays, there are too many people trying to make money or a name for themselves promoting unhelpful messages about poorly balanced celebrity weight loss programmes, or dietary supplements which apparently will help weight fall off. The role of registered and respected dietitians in the media has helped to continue to raise the profile and credibility of the profession by dispelling the many myths and unsafe practices. It is really positive to see that the BDA is rightly being used more regularly as the go-to place for the media and public agencies to ask for sound, expert evidence-based advice and interviews.

I'm sure many colleagues who worked in hospitals in the late eighties and early nineties will remember the long Nightingale wards. Two rows of beds were laid out down opposite walls with patients facing each other, curious to know more about their "neighbours," resulting in little opportunity for any privacy. I soon realised that years of studying had affected my eyesight as I struggled to walk down the length of the ward and read patients' names at the end of their beds. I would smile and lean forward, passing the time of day with whoever I thought I should be seeing, and would quickly realise I needed to be at the next bed instead awkward! Once I got my eyes properly checked, new glasses revealed a bright new world all around me and gave me the confidence needed to spot patients' names without further embarrassment.

Wooden bedside lockers were usually bedecked with vases of flowers, get well cards, ash trays and bowls of fruit or sweets. In the case of male patients, they would also usually have a urine bottle perched on one side, allowing easy access for gents to discretely hold the bottle under their bed sheets to relieve themselves without having to get up and go to the toilet. Some lockers also held secret stashes of alcohol and packs of cigarettes, tucked away by visiting relatives and friends. Back then, the wards were still single-sex and usually had a dining table or two down the middle, which allowed anyone who was able to get out of bed so they could eat and socialise normally with others at mealtimes. It was a great way to get people up and moving, talking to others and sharing news and laughter. Over the years, the move away from communal dining to save space and staff time was a backward step for many patients but I'm pleased to hear that it is now gradually returning to mainstream wards again in some parts of the UK. Each ward also used to have a nurses' desk in the middle of the ward area, allowing staff to observe patients more closely and write up their notes.

Matrons, who were generally feared as strict guardians of their areas, had their own personal offices as you walked onto the ward, and you never dared venture in unless invited. Instead, visiting staff used the general staff office next door to read case notes and to catch up about their patients with junior doctors and key staff. It was a good way of building team rapport and sharing concerns or insights about patient care over a cup of coffee and a biscuit sourced from the stock of never-ending treats left for staff by grateful relatives.

Consultant-led ward rounds were a regular feature of every ward setting. Some were daily and less formal, while other "Grande rounds" were used for teaching a variety of grades and groups of staff. It could be quite daunting seeing them all walking round each bed, discussing individual patient's conditions, any concerns about their clinical progress and developing care plans together. Confidentiality was virtually impossible as people in neighbouring beds were easily able to overhear what was being said behind flimsy curtains. Sometimes, the news being given was the very worst — a cancer diagnosis with a poor prognosis — and patients would be left very upset, tearfully waiting for a kindly nurse or doctor to come back and explain more of what the consultant had shared and what it meant for them. Many of the senior clinicians were very encouraging to their staff while others were quite fearsome if people didn't answer their questions quite right — there were certainly some real challenging characters, usually of the surgeon variety! Incredibly, staff, patients and their visitors were all able to smoke on the wards back then, whether in bed, offices or in out- patient clinics. As a non-smoker, I found the smell really off-putting and didn't like the lingering aroma that stayed on my clothes after working in some areas. The fire risk could be quite high as people had been known to fall asleep with a cigarette alight between their fingers, so nurses had to be extra vigilant. It was a few years later before separate smoking rooms and areas were created to allow people to continue indulging in their habit, although behind the closed door, they were often hidden from view behind thick smog. Various forms of alcohol also featured on every drug trolley and patients could be prescribed cans of stout, nips of whisky/brandy or small glasses of sherry to improve their calorie intake, appetite and general wellbeing. Relatives routinely brought in boxes of chocolates or biscuits and bottles of spirits, which might be given to a loved one to keep at their bedside or were sometimes donated to the ward at the end of someone's stay. Throughout the year, quite a treasure trove accumulated in the back storeroom or matron's office, waiting to be used for Christmas entertaining. Today, students and many staff will be shocked to hear that in the fortnight leading up to the big day, a side room on every ward would be transformed into a grand party buffet of seasonal hospitality. Once you'd finished seeing your patients in the afternoon, sister would pull the curtain back and encourage you to help yourself to a vast array of alcohol, fizzy drinks, snacks and chocolates of every persuasion. It was a nice change for many on-call medical and nursing staff who might normally be found in the hospital social club at lunchtime or in the evening, as the NHS didn't introduce "no alcohol" policies until the early 2000s. I never went along to the social clubs as some of the stories of outrageous behaviour were quite notorious — and many of those involved were on call for surgery and ward emergencies!

Away from the hospital site, the social life of many hospital clinicians in Sheffield in the late 80s and early 90s was focused on the big Thursday night out at The Leadmill — popular at the time with local bands such as Pulp. You would invariably bump into colleagues from any of the city's hospitals and Friday mornings were often a test of stamina and character... There were two groups of staff in most departments — those who'd been to The Leadmill, quietly sat focused on their morning cup of coffee, willing their head to clear, and those who chatted loudly about last night's TV, family stories and the weather.

One of The Leadmill group from our team was based in a brand-new building on the other side of the hospital site and she would force herself to come over first thing to check for any mail, file record cards and say hello at the start of the day. She would appear in the main office looking bright and breezy, fully made up with red glossy lipstick, even though none of us quite knew how she managed it and felt quite depressed as we struggled on through the Friday morning routines. I discovered years later that she felt as bad as everyone else but was really putting on a show. In fact, she stayed in the main office just long enough to look good and would then disappear back to her new private office, locking the door behind her and closing the blinds before lying down on the warm, carpeted floor to sleep for the next three hours; if only we'd known at the time!!

Another of our team was married to someone who worked for a local food manufacturer, so we were often used as guinea pigs for any new puddings and cakes that his company was developing. Every dietetic department that I've ever worked in has always had a bountiful supply of sweet goodies and chocolates on hand — ironic but true!

We all had a good working relationship with the catering teams — and so we should have — as eating and drinking well is fundamental to good health. Dietitians need to be closely involved in developing and coding new general and therapeutic diet menus as mealtimes are so important in helping people to recover well and get stronger more quickly. At The Northern General Hospital, bulk trolleys of food would be brought up to the wards and the nursing staff would plate it up for patients, giving them the portion sizes and choices they wanted as much as possible —very person-centred care. There were very few nursing assistants in those days, as support roles were still in the early stages of being developed and domestic staff weren't allowed to be involved in the meal service, except to help clean up dirty dishes, which were washed and stored in the ward kitchen.

The nurses were able to see clearly who hadn't managed to eat very much and could use their own initiative to make up small snacks and milky drinks in the ward kitchen — day or night — for those who needed them. Occasionally, popular choices would run out quickly or patients would maybe miss a meal when they were away for x-rays, etc., but the kitchen would always be able to provide something nutritious for them. In the newer part of the hospital, heated trolleys containing ready- plated meals started to be used on the more modern wards and were regenerated before being given to patients on airline-style trays. There wasn't the flexibility of having different-sized portions, so, on the orthopaedic wards for instance, you could have big strapping men receiving the same size portion as a little old lady. If there were spare meals on the trolley (if someone had been discharged in the morning), there was at least the potential to offer seconds. The design of the trolleys was still evolving and often meals would overheat or become very dry. Salads and ice creams would warm up and become inedible, which made it quite a challenge to please everyone, but especially patients who really needed additional nutritional support. It wasn't a popular form of providing meals and created even more problems for us on the burns unit. Calorie and protein requirements were far higher than normal due to increases in metabolic rates linked to infections, stress and to the amount of healing that was needed. Patients often didn't feel like eating much due to pain, discomfort and poor appetites which were not helped by the awful smell created by burned flesh. We had adults and children on the unit so we had to make sure that there was a wide range of choices at, and between, mealtimes. I managed to persuade Roy, the catering manager, and his deputy Denise, to provide extras like sandwiches, crisps, chocolate biscuits and a special children's menu. Often, the adults preferred to choose from the children's menu and Roy's team were happy to oblige with bigger portions, knowing what a difficult time many of them were having. Being person-centred and compassionate is what we expect for those caring for us and we must do everything we can to help alleviate suffering, menu fatigue and enjoyment of mealtimes —even in the most difficult of circumstances. The role of care caterers is so valuable and challenging but it is equally often underappreciated and inadequately resourced. Back in the eighties, the catering team also had another demanding group to keep happy — in the consultants' dining room... really! I couldn't understand why there would be a unique place for them to eat. It was a bit of an old boys' club, as there were no female consultants employed anywhere in the hospital at the time. They were served separately from everyone else by catering staff and no one could get in to use the meeting room until their lunch break was officially over at 2 pm. Even then, the air would be thick with cigarette or pipe smoke and the tables would be covered in ash and crumbs. We were told that they needed a confidential space to be able to discuss clinical cases but of course the rest of us clinicians had to make do with having lunch in the main dining room with the rest of the hospital staff and members of the public. Thankfully, those inequitable, elitist days are long gone, never to return, I hope.

Like many people in their early twenties, I started to develop more of a social conscience while working in Sheffield, so I volunteered in my spare time, working for The Samaritans once a week and occasional weekends, for a couple of years. I also started helping on Saturday morning at the large, modern Oxfam shop near my home in the west end. That gave me the opportunity to furnish my first house from the wide variety of nice second-hand goods and charity products. Both of these projects gave me a great insight into the life of Sheffield people and to chat with individuals that I wouldn't otherwise have come across. It also helped me to continue to build my confidence and skills in communicating with the public so I was disappointed to have to give it up in the end as my venture into freelance dietetics took off. It began at a local GP's practice where I was employed by a large pharmaceutical company to support patients taking part in a trial of a new lipid-lowering drug they were developing. I saw patients during clinic sessions in evenings and Saturday mornings at the practice on the edge of Derbyshire. I used a structured, standardised method of assessing the dietary changes they had managed to implement, and submitted it to the GP, who was collating a varied range of clinical data for analysis by the company's trials team. I also had the opportunity to provide dietetic advice and expertise needed to support individuals' medical treatment at the two local private hospitals in the city. A great variety of individuals, from a wide spectrum of the local population, were referred to me directly by hospital consultants and I would see them either as in-patients or in their own homes, outside my NHS working day. It was a real eye-opener for me to be working in private hospital settings, compared to what I was used to in my day job. The modern, individual, en-suite hospital facilities seemed so luxurious and the contemporary varied menus available to patients and their visitors were the envy of NHS caterers; hotel standard really. I was never quite so comfortable when arranging to see patients in their own houses as there was always an element of uncertainty about what I was going to encounter and whether others might also be there. Thankfully, I didn't have any nasty surprises and continued offering a private dietetic service during my working life in the city.

Sheffield continues to have a great public transport system and I was young and fit enough to keep up the pace of working for the NHS and as a freelancer, but I quickly realised that I would have a much better quality of life if I could only learn to drive. Once I'd made that decision, I was desperate to get on with it so I embarked on a 6-week intensive driving course with a steely determination to pass. It was the best decision I ever made and I was very pleased when I succeeded, allowing me to send off for my full driving license. It put to bed memories of a previous, disastrous, failed attempt during my time as a student back in Aberdeen. I had a near miss with another car as I attempted to manoeuvre past a double decker bus at the main set of traffic lights leading up to the very busy Holburn St junction. The examiner nearly got out of the car as the sound of blaring horns around us got louder! Even now, I can still vividly recall the experience anytime I drive through the area on visits to the city.

The freedom of independent driving is something I have continued to embrace and I have enjoyed the experience of having a variety of cars over the years. My first one was a second-hand navy VW Polo, which had no power steering, electric mirrors or the other standard mod cons of today. It even had a manual choke, which I became quite adept at using as it was quite a temperamental vehicle! My normal journey to work had previously involved a 45-minute commute across Sheffield, relying on two different buses, but having the car reduced my travelling time, kept me warm and dry and saved me from carrying heavy bags around. It also gave me so much more flexibility for my evening work and allowed me to get more easily to dietetic branch and trade union meetings in other areas of Trent.

In early 1991, I received an invite from Dr Elsie Sutherland to deliver a presentation about nutritional care of burns patients at the European Burns Association meeting in Barcelona. It was yet another great opportunity which had come from my presentation to the BBA in Wakefield. The burns team in Sheffield were very encouraging and offered to help sponsor my trip, so I happily accepted. I continued working at The Northern General until April 1991 when I was offered a promotion to become the chief dietitian in the specialist spinal injuries unit, at Lodge Moor Hospital in the southwest of the city. Sadly, it soon became clear that local funding from the burns team for my conference debut in Spain was no longer on the cards, despite the positive PR for the city that it would have brought, so I had to cancel my plans and have never yet been able to visit Barcelona. Maybe during my retirement…

I channelled my disappointment into a more positive plan and set about making a success of the opportunity to specialise in the care and treatment of people with spinal injuries. I also worked at the much smaller rehabilitation unit in the local King Edward VII cottage hospital, out in the beautiful Yorkshire countryside. Lodge Moor was surrounded by lots of flat green space and was a very calm, peaceful place to work — an ideal setting for patients' long-term treatment and rehabilitation. It offered a lovely, caring and positive environment for staff and patients despite the awful injuries that so many people had suffered. The unit was run by two very jovial consultants — Mr Ravichandran (Ravi) and Mr McLelland — who were quite the double act. They had many years of clinical experience and expertise behind them and were a mine of expertise and information about the management of spinal injuries. We saw many new patients who had experienced a variety of tragic situations and there were lots of past patients who needed ongoing support. Many had to be admitted for specialist treatment of a variety of problems and complications related to limb fitting, bowel movements and skincare.

It was quite scary to see firsthand how quickly someone's life could change and I can vividly recall seeing one woman in her early forties who had been involved in a fairly minor car crash, which resulted in a complete fracture of her c-spine. Like all new patients, she had to have complete bed rest in traction, staring up at the ceiling, unable to do anything for herself, facing life ahead as a tetraplegic. Staff tried to help by positioning mirrors or portable televisions above beds but it was often quite hard to get the angle right, and, of course, patients couldn't always change the channels themselves — not all TVs came with remote controls in those days and the signal could be quite temperamental. We are fortunate today to have such a myriad of technologies, allowing us so many more opportunities to have a far greater level of independence, entertainment and communication. ying flat on their back in traction created lots of challenges for patients who really struggled to be able to eat and drink enough; malnutrition and dehydration were real risks to their health. We struggled to monitor their progress as their muscles naturally reduced and it was difficult to check peoples' weight, even for those moving about in their wheelchairs. Once a new set of specialist digital wheelchair scales arrived, patients were able to propel themselves onto it and just subtract the weight of their cushion and chair afterwards. Our physiotherapists became quite good at recording the weights of a wide range of equipment used by patients, which made it much easier for me to help monitor and plan their nutritional care. In 1992, I decided to set up a network of spinal injury dietitians from all over England, in much the same way that the burns interest group had evolved. We organised a really successful conference in Lodge Moor Hospital, which brought lots of sponsorship and expert speakers for a full day of learning and networking. We completely took over the large gym area and shared examples of our practice, trouble-shooting challenging situations and encouraging each other to continue to network afterwards. I really enjoyed my time working there as everyone knew everyone else who worked at the hospital and it was a very friendly, sociable place to work. Staff Christmas lunches in the central dining room were much anticipated as they involved all ward areas and departments, from consultants to domestics. When the Christmas pudding was eventually carried out, a large measure of brandy was poured over the top and set alight, before the catering manager ran around the huge table with it. It looked quite dangerous, making many of us quite anxious about her tripping and the potential for burns as she sped closely past us all. I'm sure that any risk assessment now would have deemed such an activity far too unsafe but this was the early 90s and the health and safety industry hadn't quite got the same grip on the NHS as it does today. Every speciality I have ever worked in over the years made me even more cautious about suffering from the same conditions as my patients and has encouraged me to always do the best I can to raise the profile of the dietetic role in their care. My next opportunity for promotion and another change of speciality came up in the BDA jobs list during the summer of 1992.

Chapter 5 — Moving on

By the time I left Lodge Moor in September 1992, the hospital was preparing to close and move over to a new, purpose-built spinal injuries centre on the other side of the city at The Northern General Hospital. Everyone was looking forward to the new facilities but there was still a huge emotional attachment to the familiarity and peacefulness of Lodge Moor.

Around the same time, I was invited for interview at Leicester General Hospital for a promotion to the newly created role of chief dietitian, a position that involved leading their specialist renal and ITU dietetic team. To this day, I've never been through such a rigorous appointment process. It started when I was asked to complete a psychometric test, before having lunch with other clinicians from the renal unit – consultants and specialist nurses — and chief dietitians from the other Leicester hospitals. After that, I had to deliver a slideshow presentation to the panel of three, outlining how I would take forward the service, before another half hour of questions. By then, they had the outcome of my psychometric tests with them and the renal consultant asked me to score myself out of ten for resilience. I tentatively suggested the number eight. Looking down at his notes, he nodded to himself and the questions moved on to Diane Spalding, the dietetic professional head of service for The Fosse Health Trust, which covered the whole of Leicestershire. By the time I got home to Sheffield, I was completely exhausted, but the following day I was delighted when she called to offer me the post. It took a few months of commuting and weekday overnight hotel stays before I was able to relocate to the village of Houghton on the Hill on the east of the city. It was a lovely location but it was also a terrible target for thieves. In the two years of living there, I had two VW Golfs stolen from the drive, the garage was broken into and belongings were strewn along the street; screwdrivers were found hidden under a hedge at the side of the house, presumably by someone planning to break in. Never was the burglar alarm needed more!

Work on the renal unit was relentless and it was a real struggle to fit in mealtimes and adequate drinks breaks. We had five consultants running numerous clinics, research trials, a transplant unit and a constantly busy ward full of very unwell people. The haemodialysis service was the second largest in the world, which also kept the two home dialysis nurses busy. We also supported patients at two satellite renal units in Lincolnshire. It was a steep learning curve but I quickly got to grips with carrying out anthropometric measurements, which were needed for all our patients. We used skinfold callipers to measure patients' triceps, and a tape measure — always slung around my neck like a stethoscope — was essential to monitor mid-upper-arm circumferences, along with grip strength dynamometers to record any changes to their muscle strength. My general grounding in dietetics from my time in Bristol came into its own because I was now living and breathing dietary "exchanges" of different food groups. 6g and 2g protein exchanges were the essential currency for anyone having haemodialysis while 10g carbohydrate exchanges added to the complexity of life for an insulin-dependent diabetic. Combined with all that, we had to somehow translate the science of dietary potassium, sodium and phosphate restrictions into a person-centred menu plan for all our patients. If we explained it well enough, individuals were better able to follow the advice and enjoy food enough to remain nutritionally well. The strict fluid limitation for patients was the hardest aspect of life for many people coping with dialysis and the most common thing they often most enjoyed after receiving a transplant was a large guilt-free mug of tea. We take so many things for granted when we are in good health and I felt a great obligation to all of them to see how we could limit as many restrictive aspects of the diets as possible. As dietitians, we had to take account of the patterns of each person's biochemistry, and the perspectives of medical and nursing colleagues as well as patients themselves, to keep them safe and enable them to enjoy their mealtimes more easily.

I was pleased to be able to co-ordinate an update of all the diet sheets, giving our patients a bit more flexibility and freedom while keeping them well. There are many reasons why people develop end-stage renal disease and we saw a huge range of them in our renal unit: diabetes, drug overdoses or interactions, acute illness, Lupus and cancer to name a few. Life on dialysis can be harsh and uncomfortable, plus the dietary restrictions needed to prevent a dangerous build-up of chemicals in the blood are really tough for many to follow. It can result in serious complications or even death if they don't strictly adhere to the fluid targets and avoid the wide range of potentially harmful foods. So many people were waiting for a life-changing transplant and they weren't always successful, which caused great distress for some who had waited so long for a new kidney. Also, sometimes the chance to receive one was snatched from them at the last minute. One of our elderly female patients had been struggling to endure haemodialysis three times a week for several years and was given the terrible news one morning on the ward that her 25-year-old son had been killed in a car crash. She faced a truly awful dilemma as he was revealed to be a perfect transplant match for her. The outcome of a successful operation would have transformed her life and released her from the tiring rigors of dialysis; not to mention the very restrictive diet she had to follow. However, she was just too devastated to think of herself and not only refused the chance to have a transplant for herself, but she couldn't even bring herself to allow him to be a donor for others.

In another sad case, I can clearly remember one bodybuilder in his early twenties who was admitted in acute kidney failure. He was very proud of all his muscles, having spent hours every week in the gym lifting weights. Sadly, his use of drugs to enhance his looks was his undoing and he ended up needing haemodialysis, no longer able to consume the high protein diet and shakes that he had been used to, and he soon became too weak to go to the gym again. It was a sorry sight to watch him deteriorate so quickly — and too late for him to realise that he had done this to himself.

Meantime, my voluntary work as the BDA regional steward for Trent continued during my time in Leicester and I was encouraged to attend both local and national IR committee meetings. Within a year, I progressed to being elected as the youngest-ever trade union general secretary of the BDA… more of that later.

During the spring of 1993, we were given more funding to expand our dietetic team and I was able to recruit someone new. Unusually for the time he was a male dietitian. Gavin stood out to all our patients and towered over me and our teammate Jane. He was always dressed very smartly in a suit and tie and wore a strong, distinctive aftershave. Many of the ladies would ask to see " that nice Mr James", thinking he was more senior than both of us, and he thought it was very funny to play along with them, pretending to be our manager. We worked as a great team though and hardly had time to catch our breath with so much clinical work, administration and project work with colleagues across Leicester. At the time, it seemed far more common for male dietitians to progress faster into management roles than the far greater numbers of female colleagues. I don't know if it was because the men were far more ambitious and self-confident – better able to "sell themselves" at interview — or if most women just preferred to remain in clinical practice rather than take greater management responsibilities.

The emergence of sports dietetics as another career route for the profession also seemed to encourage far more men to become interested in studying nutrition and dietetics, although many of them now work freelance rather than in the NHS.

In the autumn of 1993, I travelled to Iceland for a much-anticipated and well-needed week-long holiday, just a few weeks after my dad had suddenly died at home in the north of Scotland. On the second day, while walking round Reykjavik, I spotted the sign for the city hospital. It occurred to me that I could maybe drop in and see if Karl, the microbiologist from Sheffield, was still working there. He had known that I had always been very keen to visit Iceland and said that I should visit him at work if I ever made it there. The hospital receptionist looked quite bemused when I explained why I was there, asking if she knew someone called Karl in the microbiology department. She said there was a Professor of that name and called the department to let him know I was downstairs. It was a bit surreal but ten minutes later, he arrived, all smiles, delighted that I'd actually come looking for him. He immediately thought to suggest a meeting with one of the hospital dietitians and offered me the chance to come back the next day for more of a behind-the-scenes look round. I did just that and really enjoyed seeing the hospital layout with her, finding out more about her job and learning more about the challenges for dietitians working in Iceland. They were actively encouraged and funded to attend international conferences and events and she was equally keen to hear about my working life in the UK. At one point, we stopped outside the hospital kitchen and the cook invited me to look at the food being loaded onto trolleys for the next meal. It was all very well organised, with individual portions nicely presented in ceramic containers which were easy for patients to hold and eat from. What interested me most were the very different food choices on offer; roll mops of soused herring on a bed of pickled vegetables smelled very pungent but it was one of their most popular choices and I'm sure it would have stimulated patients' senses. She escorted me back to meet Karl and I was delighted when he invited me to his home later that evening for dinner with his family. It was good to reminisce with them about their time in Sheffield and to learn more about Reykjavik and local places of interest. I enjoyed a fabulous feast of local lamb, flavoured with rosemary and lots of garlic. Even the local "golden arches" served lamb rather than beef in their famous range of burgers, due to the expense of importing beef all the way to Iceland. The cost of most things was quite eye-watering at times but it was a very memorable week, made even better because of the friendly Sheffield connection. I had also thoroughly enjoyed the chance to appreciate the work of dietitians in another country — just as I had been able to do in India — and would go on to do again during a future trip to New York state. Years later, at a BDA conference, I was fortunate enough to win a weekend break in Iceland, courtesy of a company making salt replacements, and enjoyed the sights and sounds of Reykjavik once again!

Back at Leicester General, I continued to work closely with the three other chief dietitians and Diane, planning student placements, agreeing the enteral feeding contract, and developing common clinical standards for all staff. Margaret Bullock was the manager for the other dietitians at Leicester General. She was memorable for never throwing anything out and her office was piled high with papers, leaflets and documents, to the point that it was often hard to see if she was at her desk; a health and safety risk to say the least. Alison Scott moved to join the service as the dietetic manager at Glenfield Hospital. She was a cheery, hardworking Irish woman and we soon became good friends as well as supportive colleagues. Years later, we even became first-time mums within a month of each other and have kept each other updated on our family lives and careers ever since. She now leads a larger team at Northampton General, going from strength to strength as a dietetic role model.

In the summer of 1994, I was fortunate to be one of several members of the wider renal clinical team to be given the opportunity of travelling to Vienna for the European renal conference and was delighted to be combining work with foreign travel once again. Dietetics being the small world it is, I knew that I'd be bound to bump into colleagues from the past, and sure enough, I soon spotted Val Jacob from my days of working in Sheffield. It was a great experience and, as expected, it was full of opportunities to learn, network and share the exciting developments and projects being delivered in Leicester.

Across Fosse Health Trust, there were at least three community dietitians attached to each of the main hospital sites, including Dympna Pearson who became a well-known freelance dietitian, highly regarded for her behaviour change work and training programmes. We were a huge, extended team and only able to all come together en masse for clinical development and social networking a couple of times a year. At Christmas, Diane would arrange for a company sponsor to support a huge Chinese buffet for us all, which was a great way to network and see staff from Leicester Royal and Glenfield hospitals, often for the first time. During my two years there, I learned a great deal about many areas of specialist clinical practice and budget management, and, outside of work, I enjoyed the extensive selection of curry houses around the city thanks to the large local population who had moved to the area from the Gujarat area of India. Driving around the city and surrounding areas in November, I was always fascinated by the spectacle of Diwali, with all sorts of beautiful bright lights and colours decorating houses. As dietitians, we had to work regularly via interpreters and needed to have a good understanding of the range of ethnic food choices and those special treats prepared for religious and other celebrations. We were encouraged to try them all though they were often very sweet and I found it a struggle to eat more than one, however, it was a fun way of learning! Working alongside Diane, I became more motivated to take on a new challenge managing a larger team of staff and started looking at the BDA jobs list again for suitable opportunities.

Chapter 6 — Onwards and upwards

I left Leicester in September 1994, exactly two years after I had started, to take up an exciting role as the district dietitian for Oldham, in Greater Manchester. While waiting for my house to sell, I moved into temporary accommodation during the week, returning home to Leicestershire on Friday evenings over a period of a few months. I found myself living in a friendly bed and breakfast with a lovely local family in their remote farmhouse, a few miles away from work up on Saddleworth Moor, near the village of Diggle. It's a really beautiful area to live in during the nice weather but I soon discovered that the roads could be completely treacherous in the winter months. One evening, the snow came down so fast and thickly that I had to park my car on the main road next to the fields, rather than in the farmyard. In the morning, I was stunned to see that my car had been completely submerged in snow, as a snowplough had come down the lane early on and blown everything off the road on top of it. Thankfully, I was able to borrow a large plastic snow shovel from a neighbouring house, but it took me half an hour to get it clear enough to be able to safely drive the car anywhere. Unable to phone the hospital to tell them I would be late — no mobile in those days — I was totally shocked, when I arrived an hour late, to discover that there was no snow lying anywhere! I was red-faced, damp from melted snow-shovelling and a bit frazzled, feeling like I'd already done a day's work. Fortunately, Jackie, our secretary, knew exactly what to do and I was soon back at my desk with a nice, strong mug of hot coffee to warm me up.

Living around Greater Manchester opened my eyes to many things but I was not prepared for the number of speed cameras or car thefts — even in the hospital car park! At the time, the gadget of the day was a car radio cassette unit that could be pulled out of the dashboard area and hidden away. Unfortunately, even putting it in the glove box didn't deter the thieves and on two occasions, I returned to the darkened car park at the end of the working day to find broken glass all over the seats and no radio! My car insurance premiums rocketed while I was there, as Greater Manchester had one of the highest rates of car crime — second only to London.

Like many dietetic offices of the time, our building was much in need of some TLC, being based in fairly tired-looking accommodation on one side of the large, modern hospital block. Like most NHS sites back then, The Royal Oldham Hospital was made up of a range of stand-alone buildings, scattered throughout the grounds, interspersed with "temporary" Portakabins and newer extensions. All of the clinical services were commissioned through the Director of Public Health's office in a neighbouring NHS site so I soon learned how to construct the essential business cases needed to persuade him to expand our service. Unusually for many workplaces, there were no glass ceilings in Oldham as both our chairman and chief executive were strong, female role models who really led from the top.

Money was always tight (no change there!) and innovative budget savings and/or income generation were
expected. It was hard to create and fund new roles so
the team were always keen to explore and develop
innovative ways of working. It was a period when
audit and research were being proactively encouraged
and funded by the health board, which allowed us to
successfully bid for a number of dietetic-led projects.
After a couple of years of lobbying anyone who would
listen to me, we were selected for a much-needed
modernised building upgrade, which transformed our
office and clinic working environment. It was great for
staff morale and a great way of encouraging students
to come back and work with us. We had a good mix of
young and older staff, including Wendy, Maggie, Jay,
Karen, Jo and Elaine, and then there was Rebecca,
who always had a stash of chocolate in her drawer to
keep her going – especially after Thursday nights out
on the town in Manchester! We were soon joined by
our first male dietitian, Ray Green, who later married
Diane, another dietitian from the neighbouring team
in Salford. Jackie, our secretary, was a single mother of

two teenage boys and fussed around him a bit like she would her own lads, which he played along with to a point. Like most departments, the office admin staff are central to having an efficient, happy team and we were very fortunate to have someone like Jackie who was always very flexible and willing to adapt with great patience to help us implement all our grand ideas and plans. I was responsible for negotiating and managing our Health Authority's enteral feeding contract and have good memories of working closely with our team from Abbott — John Evans and Andy Shepherd. Their national contract manager was Cameron MacDonald, a larger-than-life Scot who was good to work with and a highly respected person in a very competitive industry.

Home enteral feeding was still evolving in the mid-nineties and only involved a very small number of our patients, much like other parts of the UK. It would be several years before it became a substantial element of contract discussions and routine clinical work for community dietitians. We all enjoyed having dietetic students on placement regularly throughout the year and there were certainly plenty of therapeutic, clinical opportunities for them to learn from in Oldham. In the 1990s, dietetic departments were allocated students from universities in all parts of the UK, which was a good way of networking with many other colleagues and lecturers. I had one quite memorable experience with a mature student who was constantly struggling to juggle her placement with her childcare arrangements, and although we felt sorry for her and tried to accommodate these during her placement timetable, it all fell apart one morning. She turned up very late once again, complaining about babysitting problems, but soon went off to the wards as planned with her supervisor. Twenty minutes later, her neighbour called the office to find out when she was coming back to collect her child as she'd been expecting her to pick him up once she'd told us about the situation. When we finally tracked the student down, she seemed to think that leaving her child with the neighbour for the day was fine. Reluctantly, she set off home and sadly, not long after, had to give up her dietetic placement. I know from recent experience that we are now much more flexible and innovative in offering workable placements. It's in everyone's interests to give them opportunities to demonstrate their learning outcomes, and they don't always have to be in the office. We need to be accommodating with staff, as well as students, but it has to be dealt with on an individual basis and unfortunately, there is not always an immediate solution. As with all busy teams, the junior staff at Oldham eventually moved on to more specialist roles in other areas and it was good to know that that they'd enjoyed being part of happy, supportive group of colleagues. I still look out for their names in publications and social media commentaries, to see what good work they're now involved with. We always tried to encourage and welcome prospective staff to come along and visit the department, especially after the refurbishment. We wanted to sell the service and let them see how motivated the team was in the hopes that they'd love to work with us. One afternoon, I had arranged for a young woman to come for a look around, hoping that she might want to apply for a recently advertised role. Unfortunately, the weather was typically awful for the northwest — really pouring with rain — and when she appeared outside Jackie's office window, she was a sad sight indeed. Her bright pink hair was plastered round her head and face, mascara was dripping down her cheeks and her clothes were soaked. She actually squelched as she walked in and sat steaming in the warm office. We gave her our usual warm welcome and a hot mug of tea but I think the whole experience was too much for her and we never heard from her again.

Another unique selling point of our area was that Oldham Health Authority was one of the few areas in the UK to have commissioned a fully functioning ethnic minority team. We had large numbers of people who didn't speak any English at all — especially young women/mothers who had come over from various parts of Asia to be married and bring up families. We were glad not to have to rely on their children to translate, as it kept them out of school and wasn't at all appropriate in many situations anyway. Andrea, the manager, worked closely with us to make sure that we could help her staff to understand what we needed to get across to patients and help explain some of the more technical terms being used. The team employed local men and women from a variety of ethnic backgrounds who really helped allow the clinics to run smoothly and gave the public confidence and a more relaxed experience of the local NHS. It made everyone's lives much easier and less stressful knowing that Andrea would help us to meaningfully engage with our patients. The personal approach was also much more enlightening than Language Line or google translate, which also have their place, as I'm sure many clinicians and patients would also agree.

During my time working in the northwest, I felt very fortunate to be involved in the regional dietetic managers' group, chaired very effectively by both Margaret Gradwell, from Blackburn, and Susan Jones (formerly of my time in Sheffield), who had since been promoted to manage the dietetic team in neighbouring Rochdale. There was always a busy programme of meetings and lots of collaborative improvement work was developed with all members of our teams, taking forward best practice and BDA guidance. We linked closely with the North West and North Wales branch of the BDA too and meetings were always well supported and attended by both staff and students. I think that positive, proactive approach from managers to the BDA in both shaping and developing professional practice was a strong driver for the careers of many very able colleagues and students in the area. My time in Oldham was one of the most successful of my career and I was fully supported in everything that I did or wanted to do, by the general management team, particularly David Curtis and John Powell. It was a time of great opportunity, innovation and optimism for everyone and our team really thrived. I continued my voluntary work for the BDA – now as trade union general secretary — and I gained an advanced diploma in dietetics and continued to develop my career options. I had the chance of building my own professional skill set in a very different way during 1997/8 when I embarked on the BDA sports nutrition qualification. The Royal Oldham Hospital was situated just across the road from Boundary Park, home of Oldham Athletic Football Club (OAFC), which was in the premier league at the time. I had always had a strong interest in watching professional football so I chose to specialise in the sport for my practical project. It had a reputation for being a pretty tough course, run by leading sport nutrition experts of the day, including Karen Reid, Jeanette Crosland, Jane Griffin and Gill Horgan. I was already juggling a busy job, while "volunteering" as the BDA Trade Union General Secretary and trying to complete my extra studies. I had to spend a lot of time on the west coast train line, so used that as an opportunity to study, read papers for meetings and write up course work, etc. By the time I'd arrive back in Oldham, I was always quite weary, and one time, I stepped out of the station and walked towards the taxi rank, keen to get home again. I put my hand on the back door handle and was about to get inside when I felt a firm hand on my shoulder and the sound of a very angry woman telling me, "This isn't a taxi, that's MY husband — clear off!" That certainly woke me up and I was very relieved when a cab finally turned up to get me away from the station.

I was able to carry out my practical sports case studies at local football clubs next door at Boundary Park. The manager of the day was Neil Warnock, a very straight-talking, experienced veteran of the game. He was willing to allow me to work with the team though I mainly linked in with the physiotherapist, Alex, who was very supportive of my role and invited me to talk with the professional players and up and coming youngsters. They were full of fun and enjoyed pranks as I discovered on more than one occasion. Once, when I was invited to sit in the stand watching a match with the staff and players, I became aware that I was a bit of a curiosity to some of the older ones, who sat laughing and joking behind me. When I stood up at the end of the game, I noticed that the thick jumper I'd been wearing felt heavier at the back — only to discover that they had been gradually pouring water on it during the second half so it was soaking wet and weighing me down...there was a good reason why they often ended up sat on the sidelines rather than playing! Alex had words with them, of course, but the next time I went to work with the team, he decided to give me a bit of a shock. I had been suggesting ways that the coaches could emphasise the importance of good hydration more with players and show them how dehydrated they'd become after a match. They should weigh themselves in their underpants before playing or training and then do the same straight afterwards, calculating how much fluid weight they'd lost. I was standing talking with a couple of the young players in the dressing room before a morning session and heard Alex approaching behind me. He said, "Right, Evelyn, let's put your ideas to the test. They're ready for you now." I turned round to find all the players lined up in their underpants waiting to be weighed. A few of them were laughing at the embarrassing position Alex had put me in. Somehow, I managed to retain my professional composure and got to work, so they soon realised that this was a serious exercise. They were initially quite shocked to see just how dehydrated they'd become after their training session and many of them then started to take a more competitive attitude to hydration. They were encouraged to use either water or a branded sports drink, as premier league teams were inundated with free supplies at the time. Another day, I was invited along to observe the younger players' training session and was astonished to see that one of them appeared to have some black plastic sticking out from under his shirt. On closer inspection, we discovered that he had fashioned himself a vest from a bin liner as he was trying to lose some weight and had decided to sweat it off rather than train harder. We soon put him right and he quickly realised that he was hindering his potential playing skills by risking injury resulting from the side effects of dehydration. Many players and athletes carry around small credit card-sized "pee charts" in their wallets to check the colour of their urine when they go to the toilet — the darker it is, the more dehydrated you are — which gives a good indication that they may need to drink.

As more players and managers moved from European clubs, many of our professional sports teams became a lot more switched on to the benefits of good nutritional care for players and the positive impact for their performance. Sports nutrition became much better understood as research was published and shared. Most professional clubs now employ specialists qualified in sports nutrition, working alongside physiotherapists, psychologists and team doctors.

Unfortunately, trying to change attitudes about their diets was much more challenging for some of the older players. Many sports people can become very superstitious about following pre-match routines and have odd rituals in the lead up to a game; especially if they've previously won a match after eating a particular meal. One case in point was a player who refused to eat anything else but a large bowl of rice pudding an hour before playing a premier division game and no amount of rational discussion could change his mind. For my sports nutrition coursework, I also had the opportunity to spend time working with a young player at Bolton Wanderers F.C. My contact was, once again, the club physiotherapist – Euan — who was a friend of Alex from Oldham. I discovered that many of the first team were being encouraged by the manager to take a new nutritional supplement to enhance their playing ability. However, the ingredients bore no resemblance to anything I had come across before and I contacted a variety of sources to try and establish what they were and what value they might have for sports performance. None of my tutors on the sports course had come across anything like them either so I fed back my concerns to Euan who then introduced me to the manager of the day – another well-known veteran of the game. It wasn't that there was any question of the ingredients being illegal, but we couldn't establish any nutritional benefit either. I was left in no doubt that he wasn't at all interested in the views of any dietitian and said in no uncertain terms that the players would continue to take them as long as he was there. It was quite a contrast to what my colleague was experiencing along the motorway in Old Trafford but I continued my case study with the 18-year-old aspiring professional anyway.

It was around the time that construction of the new Reebok stadium was nearing completion so I was very fortunate to be given access behind the scenes and to attend several big matches once the club was fully functional. I continued my sport nutrition studies back in Oldham at a time when OAFC was trying to establish itself as a football academy. They were keen to support and invest in young players early on with a much more professional approach to training, using the sound evidence of the day. I was approached by Andy Gray, the club's acting manager, who asked if I would work with the boys three evenings a week after school. This new venture happily coincided with me being pregnant with my twin daughters. At the time, the only challenges I had were caused by feeling extremely tired by 1 pm most days. Working with the football academy meant that I was able to go home and sleep for the afternoon before heading out for a few hours, working with the young lads and their parents from teatime until mid-evening. Previously, the boys had been turning up for training straight from school, in many cases having not eaten anything since lunch. Often they had only eaten a packet of crisps or sweets, washed down with a very sweet orange-flavour drink, which was popular at the time. My main aim was to help all of them understand how nutrition could help them perform better, and, in a few weeks, they saw positive improvement, proving my input to have been a great success. We were able to help them to see how making changes to what they ate and drank before and after each training session and match could really help them feel better on the pitch and improve how they played. They also commented that they were now going home after playing, without having headaches or feeling ill, which meant that they were also sleeping well.

Chapter 7 — Life in the Southeast.

I left the team at Oldham in November 1998 and my twin daughters were safely delivered in January 1999; something for which I will always remain very grateful to the NHS. I felt that I'd left a positive legacy with the club, but my career took another unexpected upturn after a few months, and I never returned to find out if they continued the work that had been started. I had fully intended returning to my role after my 12-month period of maternity leave, but in the spring, I spotted an advert for a district chief 1 post being recruited for down in Gillingham, Kent and decided to apply for it. This was a rare career opportunity as many of these senior clinical management posts had disappeared during various health authority re-configurations. I was interviewed in the centre for rehabilitation services at Medway Hospital, and, walking into reception, I was confounded by a smell which was a distinct mix of wood, plaster of Paris and rubber… The building was home to several specialist support services such as orthotics, prosthetics as well as the wheelchair team. There was also a range of workshops at the back of the building, where skilled staff produced many items of equipment needed by disabled service users. First impressions were very positive and I was warmly welcomed by Jill, a friendly receptionist/cleaner/general assistant who always seemed to know everything and everyone. She ushered me through to the office of the lead rehabilitation consultant, Dr Lal Landham, who would be interviewing me alongside Lynne Brown, my soon-to-be manager.

I was delighted to be offered the post the following day and I moved south to start work at the end of July 1999. I set about putting my house in Rochdale on the market and moved to Gillingham during a particularly strong heatwave. It was almost overwhelming and so totally different from the constant rain and fog that I'd been used to up in The Pennines. House rentals were hard to come by, but I was fortunate to quickly come across one that was being renovated by a couple from Inverness and was relieved to be able to move my family in a couple of weeks later. During my induction, Lynne introduced me to staff and directors at the PCT headquarters. I met the director of finance and immediately felt the hairs on the back of my neck stand up. I knew her from somewhere but wasn't certain, until later that afternoon, it came to me. I realised that we had been to primary school together, spending hours after school playing card games with her sister, who was now her deputy director of finance! We hadn't seen or heard from each other since 1976 but soon arranged to meet for coffee and catch up. We remained friends during my time in Medway and regularly met up with our children outside work. What a small world we live in, eh?!

The dietetic team were very friendly, and I was welcomed by senior dietitian, Lois Carnie, who had been holding the fort during the period of vacancy. She was a very driven feisty Scot, who became one of the few dietitians I have known to go on to change career in the same organisation, transferring into the embryonic IT department a few years later. Use of new technology and e-communication still had a long way to go to becoming as integral to our workplace as it is today, but I was pleased to find that I finally had my own workplace computer. It was still incredibly rare for anyone to have a work laptop and my standard-issue mobile phone was generally referred to as a brick. I sent my first text on that one and recall that I couldn't even work out how to add in punctuation, so it's amazing that anyone could understand my messages! We had regular staff clinical updates and meetings which brought the whole team together to share, learn and encourage each other. Everyone was really encouraging and supportive to their colleagues and keen to develop our team further, which made my job as manager so much easier. Each department I've ever worked in has surprised me in different ways, and in one of my early team meetings, I was a bit non-plussed by an example from Gillingham. We were discussing the best way to plan staff cover over the Christmas holidays, which was going to potentially be a difficult juggling act, as so many staff had young children.

The conversation moved on to talking about working during bad weather and having previously experienced some atrocious driving conditions in both the Pennines and South Yorkshire, I was quite surprised to be even having the conversation. Lois raised a knowing eyebrow in my direction as someone asked me what my view was of "snow work". I had never come across the term before and was curious. Essentially, staff hoped to stay at home if there was any snow on the ground, using the time to catch up on CPD activities, develop recipes and other personal projects. While I am a positive advocate for homeworking – especially since lockdown — the idea just wasn't sustainable at that time as it would potentially mean that most of the team would have stayed away from work during snowy weather. If everyone had the technology that we have today, it might have been more possible, but as it was, there was a real concern that "snow work" would probably have caused the service to collapse.

Meanwhile, the enteral feeding contract was again my responsibility and, as a team, we were now starting to see an increase in the potential for more patients to receive and manage their tube feeding at home. Companies had started to employ nursing specialist roles to support patients and to train community nursing staff in this new service. The range of products was now much more extensive with improvements to flavours, presentation packaging and nutritional composition. One of the large companies started to develop the first e-registration system but it would be several years before that was fully tested and rolled out as so few staff had access to computers and lacked the IT knowledge needed to use them. Within five years, home enteral feeding became routine, transforming the care and quality of life for so many people.

Whilst working as the dietetics manager at Medway, I had the opportunity to re-structure the team and pursue my own clinical interests, knowing that I had three great team leads who were supporting me to run the service smoothly. Julie Webster, Kerry Smith and Fiona Jenkins were all very experienced, easily capable and managed their clinical teams well. There were lots of busy part-time young mums, including Anne, Jo and Lorraine, who were all hard workers and very encouraging of one another: Anne even studied for an Open University degree and achieved 1st class honours on top of her paediatric work and raising a family! Our admin staff kept us all on track — Vanessa was always "just popping outside for a quick ciggie" with Barbara from the limb-fitting team across the corridor; then came Karen who was a super-organised office manager who was also a fervent Gillingham FC supporter in her spare time. Like most progressive dietetic departments, we created roles for two dietetic assistant posts and were approved to take several student dietitians on placement during the year. However, what no one had told me when I started my job was that I was not only responsible for overseeing the placements in Medway; I was also expected to co-ordinate 32-week placements with the dietetic teams at Lewisham and Bromley hospitals in Southeast London... There was still very little in the way of email communication in the early 'noughties', so we had to use a mixture of post, phone and occasional face-to-face communication. I found it quite a challenge, given all the other pressures of my job, my lack of knowledge of driving round the southeast motorways and trying to make sure that the students could have a good experience when they were with us. There was a good network of dietetic managers in the Southeast though, and I found them very supportive and enjoyed hearing what all their teams were up to. I was pleasantly surprised to find an old face there at one meeting — Lesley, my RGU classmate, who had watched my early catering disasters alongside Jan, back at RGU. She managed the community dietetic team in Eastbourne, having started her career there straight from university, gradually working her way up through the grades to her current post. It was refreshing that she was just as I remembered her and was still as engaging and friendly as ever.

Having been very involved with the BDA over many years, I was surprised that many of my counterparts were not so used to making the most of the opportunities for support and help from our professional organisation. I'm grateful that they were quite tolerant of my enthusiasm for it –even if they were sometimes less than keen themselves. A couple of years into my post, I was able to apply for a brand new role, which had been created as part of the NHS plan of 2000. There was now a better commitment to fully engage clinicians at Trust Board level, in making strategic decisions about local NHS service re-design and governance. The creation of the Professional Executive committee (PEC), described as the "engine room" of the primary care trust (PCT), offered 2 AHPs the incredible chance to progress to hold a board-level position, with extra remuneration on top of their own salaries, to reflect the additional responsibility of the roles. I was encouraged to apply by my team, and manager Lynne Brown, and was delighted to be appointed to the PEC two days a week, with backfill for my team. The chair of the PEC was a GP who already had a busy practice to run, a personal business and other parallel work for the PCT. It soon became clear that he wasn't able to fulfil the busy role of the PEC chair without more help, so, following a discussion with the rest of the PEC- made up of 5 GPs, another AHP and 3 nurses plus our CEO and Director of Finance- I was elected to the new role of PEC vice-chair. The post took up at least half my working week and

I was given so many great opportunities to develop my leadership skill set. I took on far greater responsibilities than a dietetic manager would ever have been able to experience normally. I was able to chair the PCT finance and commissioning group and, alongside Sally, our bright bubbly communications manager, had the board level responsibility for PCT communications. My office base was predominantly in the PCT HQ — a basic, functional building in a business park on the outskirts of Gillingham. IT facilities and administrative support were fantastic, but space was limited and walls were thin, which meant we all had to be very tolerant and accommodating with colleagues and visitors on the premises. On one memorable occasion, tolerance was stretched to breaking point one lunchtime… In the small downstairs kitchen, close to the offices of the CEO and Chairman, a new member of staff made the rookie mistake of deciding to heat some kippers in the microwave! The smell met you at the front door, filtering through the two-storey building. He was met with a barrage of outraged secretaries who left him in no doubt that any future attempts at cooking should be significantly less fragrant... *and* in the upstairs staff room. Needless to say, he never made the same mistake again.

My career, however, went from strength to strength and by 2005, I had been formally elected to the post of PEC Chair — the first dietitian and only one of three AHPs in England to hold the position. It meant far more responsibility for me, as a member of the board, and I worked very closely with my Chairman and Chief Executive, in a model of working described by NHS England as "the three at the top". We planned and co-ordinated board meetings together and worked collaboratively with other teams across the Kent and Medway strategic health authority. We had fun too, during team-building events with PEC/Board and management team members, usually in the tranquil setting of Aylesford Priory. I recall one exercise where we were all trying to understand each other's personalities and strengths better when we were asked to describe ourselves as a shape — a square, a circle, a triangle or a squiggle. Not one to be pigeon-holed into anything obviously conventional, I chose a squiggle... I explained that I preferred to choose to go my own way and do my own thing, not wanting to be constrained, and able to take innovative approaches according to what I felt was needed. I thrived in having the chance to work transformationally rather than the more routine transactional, tick-box approach. They all nodded in agreement, having seen the work I was doing in my dietetic career. Board meetings invariably went on until late into the night, as there was so much innovative health care business being developed locally at the time. It was quite a juggling act being a single parent, having to make complex childcare arrangements for my daughters, who were now in primary school, and getting enough sleep. Most evenings, I was in bed by 8 pm, which caused great amusement to colleagues who couldn't understand why I wasn't able to join in conversation about TV programmes the night before. It was the only way I could survive and keep going, giving me enough energy to make the most of the time I had with my children when I wasn't at work.

The role of AHPs became much more high-profile across Kent and Medway because of our presence on the PEC and through local transformational work. Physiotherapists, podiatrists and a podiatric surgeon massively reduced orthopaedic waiting times by treating people before they got anywhere near a general surgeon, helping to keep the PCT well within the notorious waiting times targets. We were able to plan, commission and introduce new intermediate care and same-day treatment centres, which were very successful in reducing the strain on the local hospital bed and theatre capacity. It was great to be working as part of such a positive, dynamic organisation, delivering far better and faster care for local residents.

Our Director of Public Health, Anita, was a great proponent of new technology and gadgets — easily navigating the highways and byways of the Medway and Kent landscape using a sat nav, which not many people had back then. She was the first person to introduce me to the concept of Wi-Fi at home, which allowed her to work anywhere she wanted around the house while her children had their own computers, reducing the potential for any arguments about who could use hers. It was a far cry from my second-hand, clunky one at home with a huge hard drive, which connected slowly to the internet via a cable attached to the phone line. The accompanying shrieking noise as it did so was eye-watering! We take the luxury of easy access to our range of gadgets and technology so much for granted today, don't we? As a Board member and PEC Chair, I had my own office, equipped with a desktop computer, and was supported by Sylvia, my really efficient secretary. She supported me in navigating the world of office technology and I became a bit more confident using it, helped in some ways by having access to more IT training opportunities. On one such study day — the 11th of September 2001 — I was part way through an event only for it to be interrupted by someone rushing in to switch on the television news. We watched in stunned silence as the second plane crashed into the second of the twin towers in New York. One of our secretaries had a son working in a neighbouring building and we waited with her until she heard that he had fortunately escaped with his life: it was a surreal situation and certainly put our own comfortable lives into perspective.

Chapter 8 — Life behind bars

Throughout my career, it has never failed to surprise me how life can change quickly through chance meetings or conversations. One morning in 2000, I was sat working at my desk in the rehabilitation centre when I took a phone call that would change my working life for several years to come. On the other end of the line was Howard Pemble, the healthcare manager at HMP Rochester, who wanted to know what nutritional advice or support might be needed for someone who had been burned. More precisely, one of his prisoners had been targeted and scalded with a sweetened hot water mixture, which had been thrown over him in an unprovoked attack. Someone subsequently described to me that the difference between male and female establishments was that "women do drama and men do trauma!" As a former burns specialist, I was able to give him the benefit of my experience and shared some helpful tips for the man in question. However, my curiosity about this unique area of practice was piqued, and we arranged for me to visit him in the healthcare block so that we could have more time to discuss the potential nutritional needs of all the inmates. At the time, the prison was made up of several wings, one of which housed illegal immigrant detainees, awaiting removal to their home countries. Many often had undiagnosed medical problems like diabetes and some tried to manipulate the system by going on hunger strike. In the prison medical wing, there were "in-patient" cells, where these men were watched through an open door, while officers sat outside recording any fluid or food being consumed. No prisoner was forced to eat but staff would leave out bags of sugar so they could make sugar water for themselves and there were cartons of prescribable chocolate flavoured drinks to tempt them to break their fast. Once they were seen to start taking sugar or supplements, they would be returned to the main wing. There was also a sex offenders' wing, segregated for everyone's safety, away from the rest of the prison population, in a separate building . Men of all ages were housed there, convicted of crimes against both adults and children, and they were at risk of attack from others. Another rehabilitation wing housed men coming to the end of long sentences who would often be out of the prison during the day, doing work experience in local businesses, or they would have jobs on the prison farm, tending the pigs or vegetables. The two wings of young offenders housed an unpredictable mixture of testosterone-fuelled lads from Kent and London, with revolving-door knowledge of the prison system and a bitter dislike of each other. Like so many teenage lads, they were generally poorly nourished, lanky and always looking for extra food, keen to build up muscle bulk. Many were regular drug users on the outside, spending money on drugs rather than nutritious food. There were many sad cases of past neglect or abuse and a large percentage of them had had little or no formal education, employment or positive family relationships. Being in prison was often the only time they had a clear head, any kind of routine or a guaranteed mealtime, so lots of them were keen to improve their general health and fitness during their sentences.

The catering manager was a young but really experienced positive chef called Wayne, who I got on very well with, and we developed an enduring, mutually respectful working relationship. As is common in the prison service, many of the kitchen work force are prisoners, which helps to keep the running costs down. They were in a position of great trust, of course, and had to be relied on to behave responsibly and safely given the number of knives, access to boiling water and the potential to tamper with the prison food. The prison rules meant that they had to request to use a sharp knife or meat cleaver, which was kept in Wayne's office, and they were all supervised by prison catering officers. However, it was a great change for the prisoners from life on the wings because they were paid to work and also had the opportunity to study for further qualifications, which they would hopefully be able to use on the outside. The trouble with this arrangement, however, was that they never quite knew whether they were going to be in the prison long enough to complete any courses as they could be moved to another prison at any time, with little or no notice.

A large amount of the raw ingredients for food production came from prison farms, based in a variety of prison sites across England, which again kept costs down even if the produce wasn't always the best quality — think "wonky veg"! There were numerous problems with the supplies of potatoes, which came pre-peeled in big vats of preservative, causing them to have an impenetrable outer "skin". Despite everyone's best efforts, kitchen staff found it very difficult to soften them, regardless of whether they were soaked in water, baked, roasted or boiled, resulting in a large amount of waste, which would be recycled back to the pigs… In many prisons, inmates would tell officers that they were either Muslim or vegetarian in the vain hope that they could get spicy curries and the like; desperate to have more flavoursome choices. Wherever I worked over the subsequent years, prison menus were varied and, at least on paper, could have been described as "healthy." Inmates supplemented their main meals by using their own money to buy food from "the canteen" (a prison shop) which was stocked with a range of toiletries, stationery, phone cards, snacks and drinks. The choice available in them was decided by a prisoners' committee with representatives from each wing, vying with each other to meet the wide-ranging demands of their landings. Their relatives and friends were also able to buy food from the vending machines in the visiting area but anything being brought in had to be unopened, and was subject to a thorough search, of course. Staff were just as likely to be searched and I arrived at the prison entrance one afternoon, just as visitors were being checked in at the main gate. I had just been signed in and collected my keys and key chain when I turned round to see a sniffer dog appear with his handler. I was lined up in the draughty area with a mix of mothers, babies, friends and other assorted visitors and asked to stand still while an eager sniffer dog moved round us all.

Even when you know that you have nothing illegal on you, it is still quite daunting and hard not to step back when a large German shepherd starts circling you... Any clinician thinking of working in a prison environment must make sure that they know what they can or can't bring into prison for both treatment and teaching purposes. I arrived in the healthcare office afterwards, feeling slightly unnerved, but talking with Karen, the team secretary, I discovered that there had been times when baby's nappies, prams and various other unmentionables were found to contain contraband during these impromptu searches.

I was pleased that my role and further potential at HMP Rochester was appreciated and with the support of Howard and Francis Labinjo, the prison medical officer, I started working in Rochester prison each Tuesday afternoon. Initially, it started on a six-month trial basis to try and show the number one governor that there was a value to having a dietitian working as part of the wider healthcare team. As I got to know the prison staff and talked about how my job could help prisoners, I developed several roles that they found most useful. I would see individual prisoners for 1-1 therapeutic advice; I worked with groups of young offenders, talking about eating well in prison and also thinking about how they looked after themselves on the outside; I delivered presentations as part of well-being classes in the education block and on the sex offender wing, at the request of staff. I also tried to include prisoners in national health promotion initiatives that the mainstream dietetic service was delivering to the general population on the outside. One week, we ran a nutrition quiz for the young offenders and the winner received a brand-new celebrity cookbook, which he immediately took to the wing staff to be registered as one of his personal possessions. These lads often had very little of any value and he was looking forward to giving it as a present to his girlfriend once he was released. So many of the young men had had very limited encouragement or support on the outside but I found them to be very engaging, fun and keen to learn in that environment. Their attitudes were probably helped because they were now clean from drugs, well fed, keeping healthy and able to focus on themselves for once. Most out-patient sessions were held in the healthcare department and I can distinctly recall the first man I saw. He was on the sex offender's block and had diet-controlled diabetes, so he needed some help navigating the prison rules to be able to access a suitable meal choice on the wing. Anything requested from the prison kitchen that was out of the ordinary could only be provided once the prison doctor had written a formal request (I had to ask him to do this) for Wayne to action. This included sandwiches for an evening snack and any extra portions of fruit or other suitable items of food. Breakfast "packs", consisting of a bread roll, a squeezy pack of jelly and a sachet of liquid margarine-type substance, were given to prisoners, alongside their evening meals, the night before weekends or bank holidays, when staffing levels were often reduced. The theory was that they could eat breakfast in their cells in the morning when they were unlocked later than usual as they had no work duties and staff numbers were limited. Invariably, boredom got the better of most prisoners and, by morning, their breakfast pack was long gone, having already been eaten the previous evening. Unless they had their own supply of snacks from the canteen, they invariably emerged feeling very hungry, irritable and desperate for lunch.

Clinic sessions at HMP Rochester were always unpredictable with a lively atmosphere, full of banter and challenge, especially when the dentist was also running his monthly clinic for female prisoners who had to be bussed round from neighbouring HMP Cookham Wood. The women shouted to each other in neighbouring holding cells and enjoyed winding up any male prisoners or members of staff that they saw passing outside their doors. I had one memorable very near miss one afternoon when I had to place a male prisoner back in a holding cell at the end of our consultation.

The man in question was an elderly sex offender and I can remember that as I approached a cell door preparing to open it, he muttered something very anxiously. I looked more closely through the cell window just as one of the women, who was waiting to see the dentist, lunged forward and started banging on the cell door. She launched into a loud, foul-mouthed tirade at the man, which only encouraged the other women in neighbouring cells to join in! The man was terrified (I was pretty shaken myself, though I couldn't show it) but I managed to get him safely into a cell of his own just as the dental assistant appeared to see what all the noise was about. Needless to say, I never made that mistake again...

Education sessions around the prison wings were always eye-opening and I particularly enjoyed the discussions with the young offenders. They were nearly all struggling with drug or alcohol issues on the outside, so we would talk about the effects of these on what they were eating. They were always full of energy, bravado and back-chat. Most of them were trying desperately to gain weight and were keen to go to the gym as often as possible to try and build up some muscle. The trouble was that they weren't eating particularly well — a heavy reliance on junk food from the canteen and lots of "fussy eaters" meant that they often didn't have the energy to keep fit. Many of them came from pretty hard backgrounds and had had little opportunity to eat a varied diet… safe to say that fruit and vegetables did not feature highly. I was certainly able to relate to many of their circumstances from my own childhood background, living in poverty and reliant on state benefits or food handouts from relatives. We managed to organise a "give me 5" campaign, involving tasting sessions of various fruit juices and exotic varieties, even though getting them in through the prison gate was quite challenging. I quickly learned that there were many things that were embargoed or could only be used by me with close supervision from prison officers. Free, branded pens might appear quite a nice, innocuous reminder of the health promotion message that I might usually have given out to the public. However, if they had a small metal spring in them, they were a potential weapon and couldn't be given to prisoners. Blu Tack was an unexpected problem that I hadn't thought of. I would have used it to put up posters but soon learned that even the smallest pieces would be meticulously collected up on wings until there was enough to be able to make moulds of tools or keys, for instance. Drawing pins were clearly not appro-priate, so I was forced to use small pieces of Sellotape from the staffroom but only as long as I didn't take the roll away because "in the wrong hands, it could be used to bind or gag someone." After all the initial preparations, the tasting sessions nearly didn't happen as we couldn't find anything to chop up fruit into small pieces for them to try... even *I* wasn't daft enough to try and bring a kitchen knife in through the main gate! Eventually, one of the officers found a plastic one, so we had great fun as the lads proceeded to hack their way into passion fruits, pineapple and mangoes. It was so rewarding to share the experience with them and to see how much they enjoyed learning and tasting things they might never have had otherwise. There might not be any legitimate alcohol in a prison but there is always the potential for prisoners to make homemade varieties using fruits, fruit juices, potatoes — anything really — so we didn't want to undermine a great health promotion session with an opportunity to make hooch back on the wing. However, prisoners are very resourceful and sometimes it's the least obvious people who turn out to be the ringleaders, as I discovered one evening when I joined in a discussion with a group of men on the rehabilitation wing.

They were out at work all day, so the evening gave us a chance to break the monotony of their life on the wing and to talk about eating well both in and out of prison. During the course of the session, we were chatting about the benefits of 5 a day and different ways of integrating fruit and vegetables into our diets. There was the usual mix of flippant and sarcastic comments alongside genuine interest, when several men started joking with an older prisoner who was sat listening politely, smiling in a quiet, unassuming way. It didn't take long to discover that he was in fact the keeper of the current "still"! The following week, I dropped into the wing office and was talking with the senior officer who was keen to know how the session had gone. He explained that they had intelligence that there was a batch of alcohol brewing somewhere on the landing but all cell searches had drawn a blank. He pointed to a display of photos showing all the men in the block and suggested a couple of people who they had thought were most likely to be involved in it. When I pointed to the actual culprit, they were shocked beyond belief and double-checked with me a couple of times, looking at each other in stunned silence. I could only imagine what happened later that week but even if they found the hooch, I am sure it wouldn't have taken long for someone else to set up another batch once the other was destroyed.

The next time I was back on that wing was to support a new inmate who had both diabetes and coeliac disease. This is a hard enough diet to follow normally but very challenging in the context of prison rules and large-scale catering, combined with a limited knowledge about gluten-free cooking. I was able to bring in some sample packs of gluten-free biscuits, pasta, bread and a couple of boxes of flour mix through the gate, with permission from Wayne, as long as I took it straight to his office. I provided him with details of gluten-free food companies so that he could request more and asked the healthcare team to get some prescribed for him. None of this is as straightforward as it sounds, though, and it was a constant challenge to help him follow his diet. Needless to say, once we managed to get it sorted, he was moved on to yet another prison!

After a while working with the healthcare staff at HMP Rochester, I started to be invited next door to carry out diabetes reviews of some women in HMP Cookham Wood. It was quite a different environment from what I'd been used to, and somehow, the atmosphere was more highly charged. Over my 7 years of working in prisons, there was a general acknowledgement that "women do drama and men do trauma" behind bars. Audrey, the healthcare manager, was keen to have me working as part of the team but always cautious to keep me safe and ensure complete confidentiality — prisoners (especially cleaners) discretely pick up and share snippets of information from every area of the prison and are very well informed. On my first visit, she took me for a walk around the prison corridors and was showing me kitchen facilities on the wings, the dining room, visitors' area and generally introducing me to senior officers. Walking onto a new section, we were suddenly confronted by a very intimidating looking inmate — young, big muscles, with hair severely pulled back and shaved at the sides, giving her quite a threatening look. She was holding a metal jug of boiling water — evident from the steam rising from it. Clearly thinking I was an inspector or someone important in my smart suit, she barked something at me. I thought she said, "How are you?" and, half smiling, I replied, "I'm fine, thanks". She took a step closer, obviously annoyed: "I said, WHO **are** you?!" It took every ounce of nerve not to take a step back, but I managed to calmly tell her who I was and why I was there, which seemed to pacify the situation.

She turned to Audrey, sucking on her teeth, and shrugged dismissively before moving on her way, presumably to tell others that there was now access to a dietitian in healthcare. Audrey wanted me to set up a diabetes clinic, to assess inmates' food intake and their understanding of the diet and to help them navigate the canteen and prison rules, generally making sure that we could help them stay well while they were with us. Many of them were older women who had been caught carrying drugs from the Caribbean as they entered the country. They had usually been stopped at

Heathrow, before being transferred to HMP Holloway until a court appearance, conviction and sentencing. They were often serving terms of more than 10 years and would spend the majority of that at Cookham Wood unless their behaviour meant that they had to be moved on around the English female prison estate. Female prisons are not categorised in the same way as men's and adult women are housed together regardless of how long or serious their sentences might be. I continued working there most weeks, and after a few months, I was allocated a set of keys and a prison radio so that I could make my own way around the wings. I was trying to deliver health promotion sessions and positively engage with women in the dining area. The only problem with that plan was that I was completely useless at responding to radio messages, partly because I wasn't attuned to the call sign I'd been assigned, and partly because I could never remember to use the correct responses when replying to any that I had somehow managed to hear. One morning, while I was sitting in one of the lounges with a group of women, talking about their experiences of prison food,

there was suddenly a huge commotion outside and 3
prison officers rushed in. The first one in the door was
a huge man, looking quite red-faced and very anxious.
He stopped abruptly in front of me and asked if my
radio was working as I hadn't responded to the routine
radio checks throughout the morning, so they were
worried for my safety. He was less than impressed
to find out that I'd turned the volume down so that I
could concentrate on listening to what everyone was
saying in the room! On another occasion, I was in a
small teaching room with 10 inmates, discussing the
challenges they were having with eating well in prison
and how life differed in the various other establishments they'd been to. This time, I had no radio as I
had been escorted there by one of the healthcare staff,
who had left me with the women while she went off to
see someone in the segregation area. We had talked
for more than an hour, so when the session finished,
I sent them off to head back to their cells: another
big mistake! As if prisoners would happily go back to
their cells when they could be wandering or skipping
along the corridors having fun! I was confronted by a

furious senior prison officer wanting to know who was responsible for the ensuing chaos, but needless to say, I had no idea what I had unleashed, and Audrey took a lot of flak for letting me loose on the wing. Fortunately, she was happy for me to continue to deliver a dietetic service and health promotion sessions in the prison during my time working in Medway. In all the prisons I've ever worked in, I can honestly say that ones where I felt most at risk were female establishments: give me male lifers any day! To give you an example in point, I was asked to visit the segregation block in Cookham Wood one morning and was closely escorted down past the cells by a rather burly prison officer. A new inmate had recently been transferred from the secure Rampton Hospital in the East Midlands and staff were very concerned because she had very poorly controlled diabetes. Her blood sugar measurements were very high, putting her health in real danger, but worse still was that this was also causing her unpredictable, aggressive behaviour, creating real risks for the safety of others. The main problem was that she was able to freely buy and consume large quantities of sugary, fizzy drinks from the canteen and no one could stop her. I questioned whether staff couldn't simply restrict the diet she was accessing but was informed that prison rules didn't allow officers to take direct action because she had capacity to know what she was doing; they simply had to try and contain the effects of her actions.

So, essentially, my job that day was to try and persuade her about the benefits of following a low-sugar diet and to see if there was anything we could arrange that would help her to take her health more seriously. We entered her sparsely furnished cell with the officer cautiously stopping at the end of her bed ahead of me. I noticed that he was slowly and deliberately keeping our arrival low key, letting her know who I was and why I had come to see her. Her large figure was covered over by a prison-issue blanket but she slowly removed the area around her head, turning menacingly on her mattress to stare towards us. Her eyes were dull and uncommunicative as I introduced myself again and attempted to start a conversation about her eating habits. Suddenly, in one swift, sweeping movement, she discarded her blanket and pulled herself towards the edge of the bed. The officer stepped forward and muttered something to her like, "It's okay, *Jacqueline,*" while simultaneously signalling to me behind his back to get out of the cell quickly. He told me afterwards that the last time she had done that she had viciously attacked one of the nurses, so they were taking no chances with me. I felt a mixture of relief and disappointment at not being able to spend more time for her but left some written information for the prisoner and segregation staff to refer to. I doubt very much that anything much changed while she was there, although it wasn't long before she was considered too high a risk to everyone around her and she was soon back in Rampton. It is hard to step back sometimes, when you think you can help someone, but I always trusted the officers and healthcare staff around me much more than my own judgement, as they always knew the inmates far better than I ever would. My work with HMPS in Kent continued to develop and I took a call one day from the No 1 governor at the high-security, category B HMP

Swaleside on the Isle of Sheppey. We had previously worked together at Rochester prison and he had been impressed by the work that I had been doing with Wayne and Howard throughout all wings, with the various groups of prisoners. He explained that there was general unrest with his current inmate population, all of whom were serving very long sentences, and officers were concerned about the potential for rioting. I could only imagine how poor the food must have been there as he went on to describe the role he wanted from me as "to keep the roof on the prison"! It became clear that the standard of food was not great, partly due to the limited budget and poor choice of produce coming to the catering manager from the prison farms and suppliers, but he was willing to invest in an improved choice of mealtimes and snacks. I had a loose plan for assessing the situation and headed over the Sheppey Bridge one morning to spend a few hours with Mick, the head cook. I chatted with various prisoners and kitchen staff to help me come up with a range of recommendations that might help to improve the situation. Mick showed me around the main areas, and we waited for the lunch trolley to arrive on one wing, only to be confronted with several angry inmates, complaining bitterly about the food they'd been given. One thrust towards us a plastic plate containing a wedge of pizza covered in congealed cheese. Mick, who had heard it all before, explained, with little in the way of compassion, that the man hadn't bothered filling in a menu the day before so had ended up with the leftovers for lunch to keep him going until teatime. He stormed off back towards his cell, supported by swearing and aggressive body language from others who'd found themselves in a similar situation. They had all become so fed up with the poor food that they couldn't be bothered formally complaining anymore and the situation had been brewing for several weeks.

We soon came up with a new four-week menu cycle with a much more varied choice of dishes to suit all the religious and cultural needs of the diverse prison population. When I visited a few weeks later, the No 1 governor had followed through with more funding and it was great to see how much things had improved.

At the lunchtime servery, prisoners were queuing up to fill their plates with a far nicer choice of well-presented food. In addition to puddings, there were also mangoes to improve their fruit intake, rather than the hard pears or sour apples of old when there had been nothing more ripe or exotic. The mood among the men was much happier and the chat was now full of jovial banter rather than grumbling complaints. Prisoners whom I had been seeing in the healthcare clinic shouted out their approval, and even Mick managed to appear content with the situation. He retired a few months' later on a high note after many years working for the prison service and the governor was very relieved that the roof was still very much intact!

Unusually, for all the prisons I visited, I was occasionally asked by healthcare staff to see prisoners on the wings when their mobility and general condition were giving cause for concern. In one instance, I visited an elderly man who had longstanding respiratory problems and was struggling to eat enough as he was gasping for breath so much. His weight had plummeted and staff needed me to see if I could offer more practical advice suited to him and then liaise with the kitchen to make sure that he could have a more varied, personal choice. As luck would have it, his son was also serving a long sentence on a different landing and was allowed to help collect food for his father from the servery, along with any additional orders from the canteen. It was agreed with officers that he could join me to meet his dad in his cell and see if we could all come up with a better plan to try and improve his condition. It was a bit of a surreal situation, and it was quite touching to see his son frantically fussing around trying to tidy the surroundings so that I could sit closer to him on his rather rickety bedside chair. I'm sure you can imagine that the smell of a male prison is something to behold — a combination of a stuffy, airless environment, body odours, stale cigarette smoke and smelly socks or dirty washing lying around — and I was sat right in the middle of it! The old man was quite a sorry, emaciated sight and he really struggled to communicate because his breathing was so bad. However, we eventually agreed a few options for snacks and meals and I headed off to agree how to implement a plan with the health and catering teams.

At HMP Swaleside, we also found ourselves in the unique situation of having to care for another elderly prisoner who had been recently discharged from Medway Hospital following a stroke and now needed to receive PEG feeding using a specialist feeding pump. At the time, it was completely unheard of to be delivering such complex care in any prison within the large Southeast prison estate, but without it, he would have died. He was quite immobile and confined to his cell most of the time, due to some difficulty in negotiating his way around in a cumbersome wheelchair. Arranging the artificial feed for him took quite a bit of negotiation between custody and healthcare staff to support his care. The nurse from our enteral feeding company helped by training the prison nursing staff to use the pump, and in arranging secure delivery of his feed and supplies. One of the biggest challenges for him was that strict prison rules dictated that cell doors could not be unlocked outside of mandated hours without great difficulty and only after navigating the internal HMP command structure. This meant that even if the feeding pump alarmed during the lock-down period, the prisoner would have to wait for wing staff to receive permission from a governor to unlock him and allow someone from healthcare to re-set the pump for him. I wasn't totally surprised to learn that a few months later, he was rushed by ambulance to Medway Hospital one morning, having apparently suffered a further stroke during the night, and he had passed away peacefully outside prison walls. I was, however, glad that we had managed to break down organisational barriers and show other establishments what could be done if prisoners ever required tube feeding in future.

Soon after, I was delighted to have successfully managed to bid for funding from the centre for health-care innovation to develop a local prison initiative, which was aimed at improving care for prisoners living with diabetes. I continued working with Sue, Dermott and others in the healthcare team to set up lunchtime training events for staff on a range of related topics. We managed to arrange to have a variety of company reps come in and showcase their products –insulins, testing strips, foot care products – and included relevant NHS staff from Medway Hospital to build stronger links with the prison healthcare team. The work was really well evaluated by staff who had limited access to company sales updates and courses and it was good to hear that this work had resulted in a positive benefit to the care of prisoners. The project was nominated for a prison healthcare award by HMP/DH staff, which resulted in Sue and I being invited to a ceremony in London during the summer of 2003. I was presented with an award for "outstanding effort in prison healthcare" from none other than the Director General of HMPS, Phil Wheatley. I had to make an off-the-cuff acceptance speech to a packed room of people and was so full of adrenalin-fuelled nerves that I have very little recollection of the whole event but everyone seemed happy with it. It would be the first of several award-winning experiences to come in my career, which I remain proud and honoured to have received. Unless you try, you'll never know whether your good idea might succeed, and unless you share what you've done with others, you'll never know what a difference your work has made in encouraging others to do the same. This recognition encouraged me to keep innovating and pushing back boundaries, making a positive difference to the various services and patients around me in the future. There was also a snowball effect, which I had not anticipated, but I can look back and see that others were watching and wanted to link my insight and experience with work they were taking forward…

Quite out of the blue, I received a phone call, asking if I would be interested in joining a multi- agency SE England prison health innovation network, chaired by David Sheehan. The work was generally aimed at improving prison healthcare provision and to share good practice extensively across HMPS establishments in England. At the time, the prison service was paying local trusts and independent contractors (GPs and dentists) for any external specialist input which made services and expertise very variable and inconsistent across the prison estate. My role in the Medway and Swale prison was very unusual and I was keen to demonstrate the benefit of good nutri-

tional care to help encourage other prisons to recognise the positive impact of involving AHPs as part of
their wider healthcare teams. It was suggested that
I might want to apply for a bursary to participate in
the first-ever international prison health study tour,
which was being jointly sponsored by The Nuffield
Trust, HMPS, DH and The Centre for Innovation. The
"prize" at stake was the opportunity to join nine other
people on a multi-agency, prison healthcare contingent, on a high-level fully funded trip, visiting a range
of New York State Dept Correctional Facilities. There
were dozens of applications from across England,
but after a gruelling interview process at The Nuffield
Trust offices in December 2003, I was delighted to be
selected as one of the ten successful participants and
I set about making plans to travel to the States with
the rest of the group in January 2004. I love the idea
that you can explore the world as part of doing your
day job and it reminded me of the opportunities I had
been able to enjoy in my travels to India, Iceland and
Austria as a dietetic specialist. It's not just about being
in the right place at the right time; it's about taking the

opportunity to promote your role and added value alongside other clinical staff. I encourage all care staff to know your worth and be confident enough to put your head above the parapet. If you don't, you may miss the chances waiting on the other side for you. Our contingent met up at Heathrow airport one very cold wintry morning and I managed to break the ice as I hauled my over-size suitcase towards them all. I had no idea what I might need to take with me, so I definitely over-packed. They thought it was quite amusing to see me struggling to wheel it behind myself and it created the chance for some light-hearted small talk to help me get to know them all. We were accompanied by David, along with representatives from the Centre for Health Innovation, DH Prison health team, HMPS and HMP Inspectorate. As we prepared for our journey, I enjoyed finding out a bit more about my travelling companions. There were 2 GPs from Yorkshire — both of whom provided medical services to local prisons — a pharmacist, 2 nurses, a psychologist, an NHS manager, and the healthcare manager from one of the more notorious London prisons. We were all keen to get there, to meet our US counterparts, learning about best practice and to see projects of particular interest, such as their successful, widespread use of telemedicine, which was not yet routinely available in the UK. I was quite naive about it all, I suppose, and the level of access we were going to have to US prisoners hadn't quite sunk in. It took several days before I fully appreciated the exclusive access and high-level collaboration between HMPS and the NY Dept for Correctional Facilities. We were to travel across NY state from the west to the east, finishing off our week-long, eye-opening, truly incredible visit by touring one of the 13 prisons on the notorious Ryker's Island. We arrived safely and uneventfully at JFK airport and boarded a waiting minibus, which eventually took us to our first hotel in the state capital. Our first morning in Albany dawned and we were escorted by senior staff from NY State Dept of Correctional Facilities for our first exposure to the US prison healthcare system. We visited a high security prison hospital facility, housing all manner of inmates brought in from a variety of prison settings to receive specialist complex care that couldn't otherwise have been delivered in their usual healthcare facilities. None of us knew what to expect when we were met at the entrance to "the ward" by armed security officers, who only allowed us in once all passports and official paperwork had been checked and noted. Floors and ceilings were all specially built with heavily reinforced concrete and materials, to minimise any opportunity for escapes from any direction, and all prisoners were strictly segregated, supervised and cared for in single rooms. There was no chance of any of them meeting each other or the potential for rival gang members to come face to face.

Later that day, we headed back east to stay in a very comfortable Manhattan hotel, which would be our base for the remainder of the trip. Our minibus took us off for daily adventures to a variety of correctional facilities over the coming week. These included Coxsackie maximum security correctional facility, which contained one of five regional medical "hub and spoke" units in NY State, serving several neighbouring correctional facilities containing a higher level of specialist healthcare services. It was fascinating to hear about their hospice facility which employed trusted inmates to help provide care for their fellow terminally ill and elderly prisoners. Another day took us to one of the most famous correctional facilities in the world — "Sing Sing". At the time, it was the oldest active prison in the US and was very proud to be running a variety of novel mental health programmes, which our GP colleagues were keen to understand more about. We were wide-eyed with curiosity as we were escorted round to visit several wings so that we could talk with guards about the work they did — not to mention their challenges — and they were happy to show us how to manage prisoner movement by controlling the sliding cell doors individually and collectively. It was virtually impossible for prisoners to have any degree of privacy though, as each cell door was made of open bars and was exposed to anyone passing by along the landing, so, they routinely hung towels or clothes up to try and make the best of it. We were also somewhat star-struck when we were told that we'd be able to visit "The honour wing," made famous in a well-known Humphrey Bogart film.

Bedford Hills was a maximum-security prison for women, and we had the chance to speak with some inmates in both their mother and baby unit and an innovative guide dog training programme, "Puppies Behind Bars", which was run by women who were nearing the end of long sentences. It was humbling to watch and listen to their experiences, giving us lots to reflect on and share back in the UK afterwards.

The next day brought new opportunities for us all — a visit to one of the most infamous, highly guarded facilities in the state. We couldn't quite believe that we had been granted special permission to go into one of the 13 prison facilities on Ryker's Island, the "Anna M. Kross Center," to learn specifically about their effective suicide prevention programme. The GPs on the trip were keen to understand how the American system managed to keep incidents of suicide or self-harm so low compared to England. We soon learned that in NY State, they considered it a major failure of the system if any attempts succeeded, so there was a very robust approach to identifying potential risks. The motivation for this concern was driven by a need to prevent any litigation from relatives for these, and amazingly, the incidence of suicide in NY State correctional facilities was actually less than in the whole of HMPS in England at the time we visited.

After being held in our minibus for a lengthy security and passport check, we were full of anticipation to be allowed to drive onto the island. Huge, burly prison guards walked us through the incarceration process from the admissions gate and on to see what cell life looked like. The reality check started quickly as we observed the conditions for a group of prisoners who were waiting for processing in a large holding cell. It was a large, foreboding area, surrounded by bars, "furnished" with narrow fixed benches around the inner edge and it had, a small shared "toilet" in the corner, with no privacy for anyone using it. Walking past, I was reminded of the last time I had visited a zoo as we were directed by the guard never to go within the yellow perimeter line painted on the brown floor. That was just far enough away from any potential attacks by prisoners with long arms who might take a dislike to either us or the staff. Each of us had the

211

opportunity to observe and listen in to initial conversations between new detainees and healthcare staff while they completed their standardised admissions paperwork, which was designed to alert them to anyone who might be considered a high suicide risk. They were not immediately merged in with the general prison population but were held, under closer supervision, until they were considered stable enough to join a wing population. We moved through the facility, following guards who were equipped with radios, pepper spray and something looking not unlike a taser. We wandered into one block, under the watchful eye of guards, who were standing within an observation room, surrounded by thick, cloudy Perspex. There were also surveillance cameras to allow them to keep an eye on inmates' movements and behaviour inside, but our "tour guide" acknowledged that there were always going to be blind spots. Moving further into a huge dormitory area, we saw that it had about 30 beds, set out in a back-to-back layout — 15 on each side.

Following in behind me, one of our very experienced, apparently unshakable UK prison inspectors gasped and let out an expletive-filled groan. I stopped momentarily to take in the reality of how these men were living, trying to remain calm, and considered how daunting it would be for any new detainee being moved in for his first night. I realised with some concern that even my colleague –thick-skinned and battle-hardened from years in the UK prison system — was showing all the signs of someone who wanted to turn and run.

Prison guards had few lines of defence if attacked even though they routinely carried pepper spray. But when violence escalated and alarms sounded, we saw groups of guards running through corridors wearing riot gear suits with helmets and padded clothing, looking like American football players, and they were invariably carrying large wooden batons. It made our UK prisons appear far less intimidating than any of us remembered.

These were not what we would call jails in Britain as the US definition of a jail is where people are held for sentences of up to 100 days. We didn't visit any of these, but during some time off, the driver of my "red bus" tour later pointed out the notorious NY jail known as The Tombs — it looked very intimidating, even just driving past. Correctional facilities hold people serving sentences that are longer than a year and who do not warrant detention in a federal prison; we were all very impressed by how extensively resourced the health care facilities were. To avoid the need to take prisoners outside the facility, they had invested in state-of-the-art diagnostic and treatment services, renal units, oncology centres and end of life care wards. We were informed that much of this investment was needed to prevent the potential for litigation, as inmates couldn't just choose to go anywhere else (regardless of whether they/their insurance companies could/couldn't afford it) and in-patient stays on the outside were only in very exceptional circumstances. The result was specially built prison healthcare hubs, where a large healthcare facility could deliver highly specialised care and clinics with input from visiting expert clinicians. We saw firsthand how inmates were bussed there for appointments, including dialysis, chemotherapy, radiography examinations and a variety of other diagnostic and treatment services.

The US Department for Correctional Service pays very close attention to any of the signs linked to gang affiliations of inmates, ensuring that rival gang members didn't end up in the same waiting area. The consequences of not knowing or recognising this were well known and staff meticulously recorded and shared lots of intelligence about this — for obvious reasons. We were certainly very impressed by how they tracked potential trouble between gangs to reduce risk of violence and it reminded me of the rivalries between the Kent and Feltham lads in HMP Rochester — on a much smaller scale, obviously! With my dietetic hat on, I was also keen to understand how catering systems differed to what I had come to know from my extensive travels around prisons throughout the SE of England. At the HQ of NY State corrections, I was informed that each of their establishments offered the same choices at every mealtime, and in their store ("canteen") each day of the year. All menus had been developed with a dietitian and offered a well-balanced nutritionally adequate choice to meet most peoples' requirements. Separate arrangements were made for people who needed specialist therapeutic diets. The rationale behind this was to discourage litigation and to deter inmates from trying to find a way of getting moved to another facility where food choices might be rumoured to be better. There were little or no exceptions to the daily menu, so if you were a fussy eater at the start of your sentence, it didn't last long!

Back at work in Kent, colleagues were fascinated to hear all about the trip and I wrote several articles about my perspectives in a number of national publications. Very few, if any, dietitians in the UK were as immersed in prison healthcare as I had become but I'm pleased to say that that is changing. I always felt that it was good to raise awareness of developing dietetic roles and services, exposing them and encouraging colleagues to emulate them in their geographical area. Writing reflectively is something that I've continued throughout my career, as I find the process quite relaxing, but it also gives me and my current area of professional interest a public voice. It took me a few months for the buzz to die down but later that summer brought more reason for celebration when I won the Kent and Medway Health Innovations Award for my work in addressing health inequalities throughout the SE prison estate.

I arrived for the awards ceremony having been short-listed to the final three in my category but was completely stunned to hear my name being announced, and I stumbled forward through the large crowd to receive my award from Christine Beasley, England's chief nursing officer at the time. Little did I know that we would go on to work more closely together in a future role. Throughout the year, I continued working on various projects, trying to improve and raise awareness of prisoners' nutritional care and promoting the opportunities for NHS colleagues to engage with HMPS.

By 2005, I was excited to have the chance to start a one-day-per-week secondment with The Dept of Health prison health team, reporting to Dr Mary Piper. The team, which was managed by Richard Bradshaw, was part of the National Offender Management Service

(NOMS) and was based at Wellington House, near Waterloo Station. We had close links with HMPS senior ministers and staff, given the challenges of meeting the health care needs of the men and women serving sentences in a very diverse prison population. I was encouraged to visit prison healthcare teams around London and, one morning, I had the opportunity of visiting the healthcare team at HMP Holloway. I was keen to understand, by talking informally with both staff and inmates, how the dietary needs of women were being delivered. I arrived early but was stopped abruptly in my tracks when the gate officer informed me that someone had been found dead in their cell an hour earlier — an apparent suicide — so I was kept waiting until the immediate emergency had passed, allowing the healthcare manager to come and escort me around. The atmosphere was tense to say the least and women on the affected wing were clearly feeling quite upset but they were open to telling me about their lives there. The nursing staff obviously knew many of them well and showed genuine care and concern for everyone's needs and feelings. I also managed to spend time finding out more from the catering manager and observed the midday meal service, which appeared to be mainly based around sandwiches, packets of crisps and a piece of fruit for pudding. The "canteen" system was organised the same way as the other prisons that I'd worked in and there was a strong focus on supporting both mental and physical well-being. Prisoners were serving sentences varying from a few months to the most severe lifers, which could lead to quite a bit of friction and drama. Many of those being held on remand at Holloway would subsequently transfer down to HMP Cookham Wood in Kent, or to one of the other female prisons around the country, once they'd been sentenced. I was keen to make the most of my time with them and understand more about the variation of their experiences. The issues and challenges involved in "keeping the roof on a prison" are many and varied, which meant governors were never going to please everyone. I came to know and work well with Alan Tuckwood, the head of HMPS catering and physical activity services, as we were both keen to improve standards of nutritional care and well-being for inmates. He invited me to meet at his offices in Corby where we discussed the potential to share learning from our successful work in several Kent prisons. In the autumn of 2005, he also invited me and my DH colleague, Sara Moore, to speak at a national event for PE instructors. Prison gyms are very popular as inmates focus on body-building and self-improvement, which meant that the staff – much like sports physiotherapists — were well placed to have a strong influence on improving their knowledge of eating well, while supporting their fitness regimes. Sara had had great success in promoting physical activity in some prison settings and we enjoyed our day delivering a double act to a packed auditorium of PE staff. I was asked to be involved in a review of prison catering by the national audit office and was invited for interview.

My extensive experience of prison catering in the SE prison estate over several years was helpful but other aspects of the prison regime also had a bearing on the evidence I gave. Yes, it was possible in theory for prisoners to eat 5 a day, but the variety and quality of produce had to be good. Breakfast packs and access to specialist diets could be improved and made more nutritious. We couldn't do much about the food in the canteen as it was the prisoners who determined what was available — not always "healthy choices" – or what relatives brought in. Practical education and tasting sessions were popular and could influence the diets of inmates — certainly on the outside — if they could access the food choices in the prison menus. There was no plan to develop a standardised catering system for the English prison estate, such as the model we'd encountered in the States, so it remained the respon-sibility of local prison catering managers to work with what they had and encourage them to engage with other departments in the same establishment — healthcare, education, and physical activity —to understand and respond to local need.

Until the NHS formally took over responsibility for prison health during 2005/ 2006, there was lots of inconsistency in the resources and clinical approach to the management and support of conditions such as diabetes. Many of the services were delivered by local

GPs who were contracted to deliver clinic sessions, but involvement of dietitians or diabetic specialist nurses was very inconsistent and sporadic. I applied for and was successfully awarded a £1500 grant from the Centre for Health Innovation and arranged visits to every healthcare team in the Southeast establishments, both male and female. I prepared standardised information packs with links to a range of evidence-based materials from Diabetes UK, etc., and delivered face-to-face sessions to healthcare staff. Use of the internet was still very limited even then, so it all had to be provided in hard copy. I was very fortunate to be able to do all this as part of my substantive post and used the grant funding to back-fill my clinical time in the dietetic department. I was very confident in the three team leads — Kerry Smith, Fiona Jenkins and Julie Webster — who developed their own management and leadership skills as well as those of their staff during the remainder of my time working in Medway. They all went on to more senior posts and Kerry continues to have great success as clinical services manager in Kent.

Chapter 9 — The cabinet office leadership programme

In support of my influential, evolving role on the PEC and PCT Board, I was nominated by my chairman and chief executive for a much-sought-after place on the 3rd cohort of the Government's Public Services Leadership Scheme (PSLS). I was delighted to be accepted but, at that point, it's fair to say that I didn't fully understand the significance of what lay ahead. It would be months later before I fully realised the extensive opportunities and the access to national agencies that the course would allow me. It was a 3-year programme, organised and run by the cabinet office, to develop staff leadership skills and potential working across all areas of the civil service and public sector bodies. It consisted of several residential sessions with regular presentations from high-pro-file speakers, an interchange placement in a complimentary national location, and great mentoring, all of which were interspersed with a variety of workshops and visits. The introductory 3-day event was in a residential setting in Ross-on-Wye and I walked into the room feeling very apprehensive, not sure what I was letting myself in for.

Our facilitators, including Janet Waters, were very used to running leadership training within the civil service and immediately inspired us with their enthusiasm, organisational skills and encouragement. Our cohort consisted of people from DEFRA, DH, The Treasury, the Highways Agency, the Warship Support Agency, the DFID, the NHS, Police and Defence procurement to name a few. One of our first activities involved being split into four groups and sharing one thing about each other that none of the other groups would guess. They were shocked to learn that one of us had been the trade union general secretary for a national organisation and, because I looked and appeared very quiet, none of them guessed it was me so it was a good ice-breaker! Despite my initial feelings of being out of place, I soon discovered that I could hold my own, which was a transformational, empowering, enlightening time in my career and I looked forward to meeting up with them all each time. The unfolding programme of speakers and leadership activities that we were exposed to was so inspiring that I sometimes had to pinch myself to believe that I was actually part of something so special. I celebrated my 40th birthday with them all during one of the Network Learning Events (NLE) and we shared all the ups and downs of life as trusted old friends. We were sub-divided into smaller Action Inquiry Groups (AIGs) and had a facilitator attached to encourage us to plan visits to new environments, which would otherwise have been quite impossible for us. We had had a great group consisting of: Trevor (DEFRA), Bob (Warship Support Agency), Karen (GCHQ), Jane (DFID), Chris and Leisl (Defence Procurement), Caroline (NHS) Paul (HM Treasury) and me (NHS). Our group motto was "challenging, supporting, learning" and we strived to create the best/most unusual/memorable experiences of any of the wider PSLS cohort. At each NLE, other groups were really impressed with what we'd been doing and where we'd been going for our AIG meetings. Bob arranged for us to have one within HMS Dartmouth in Portsmouth; another was held at NHS Trust HQ in Surrey, and I managed to arrange a trip behind the bars at neighbouring HMPs Cookham Wood and Rochester! The others couldn't believe that I would be allowed to take them into one, never mind two **actual prisons** and it created a real buzz amongst the group in the build-up to the big day. I had developed a strong, trusting relationship with the senior staff in each prison and Ed Tullett, the governor at HMP Cookham Wood, was more than happy to talk with us all about his role and even agreed to personally show everyone round the site. There was a mixture of excitement, curiosity and fear in the air as we stood in the waiting area at HMP Cookham Wood gate one morning. I had warned them all to take as little with them as possible and to be prepared to leave their mobile phones in the lockers. Ed came to escort us over to the meeting room for some introductions and to describe what he had planned to make the tour quite special. The sound of the keys and clanging metal doors is quite intimidating to any visitors and the close proximity of female prisoners wandering nearby on gardening duties was quite a revelation to them. I don't know what they were expecting but they soon settled into the visit and started firing questions at Ed as we set off to see women doing a variety of jobs in the workshops, education area and passed the relatively new young offenders area. Just a few weeks previously, I had been caught up in a real prison mini-riot as one of the young women had a serious melt-down in the recreation area, properly throwing chairs and stuff around. For my own safety, I was locked in the staff observation office by the senior officer, and watched it all unfold through the reinforced glass. The staff handled it all very professionally of course and talked her down — by now she had broken down in tears — and calm resumed as she was led away to an interview room.

I was "let out" and asked to hand out the sandwich lunches to everyone else who had been locked in their cells. It was surreal to be negotiating sandwich fillings and flavours of crisps with a wingful of young women through door hatches. Fortunately, everyone got what they wanted and I retreated back to the main prison... and some better behaviour.

I mentioned none of this to my AIG colleagues, saying only that they were a very unpredictable group and that I far preferred to work with male lifers who usually settle quickly into the routine of their long sentences. I remember how impressed the AIG all were as they listened to Ed talking passionately about the responsibility of prison staff to support, listen to and rehabilitate prisoners. I don't think people generally see prison officers as having such a caring role; certainly not in the same way that NHS staff are viewed. However, they are dealing day to day with so many damaged individuals who often have challenging social care, educational and family backgrounds. These are often made more complicated by the effects of substance misuse, abusive relationships and poverty thrown into the mix, resulting in many troubled and extremely vulnerable people. These days, there is a far better understanding of adverse childhood experiences (ACEs) and the impact of personal trauma but it is still evolving in terms of supporting troubled inmates. Once in prison with access to healthcare, psychotherapy and educational support, they are often keen to improve their health, knowledge and job opportunities on the outside. Ed proudly described some of the work being done by forensic psychologists working with staff and prisoners from the healthcare department before leaving us to continue our usual AIG meeting over lunch.

Afterwards, we headed over to HMP Rochester and stepped through the huge wooden entrance into the draughty "gate area" where I was pleased to see that the admitting officer was Dave, a jovial person with the kind of wry outlook on prison life borne out of many years of experiences in the service. He checked us all in and handed me my keys, belt and chain, which I'd been trusted to wear for most of my time working there. Howard Pemble, the healthcare manager, came over to welcome us all in, pleased that I had wanted to invite them all to see round the accommodation. The AIG walked round with a degree of disbelief as they came into close contact with prisoners on the wings and as they walked through the grounds. It often surprises people when they hear how much work and responsibility I had in the prisons but it came down to strong, trusting relationships and a mutual appreciation of our joint responsibilities and attributes. Howard went ahead and opened doors to each wing while I followed behind locking them, which the others wanted to know more about — naturally, my lips were sealed as I had been warned by a security officer, early in my prison career, to "never discuss the keys". The rest of our PSLS colleagues and lecturers were amazed and maybe a bit jealous to hear all the stories from our day behind bars; a first for the programme but hopefully not the last.

The standard of our access to more high-profile areas of government started when our introductory AIG visit had been organised in September 2003. Pinching myself and drawing a deep breath, I had found myself across the road from St James's Park, walking up the steps of the HM Treasury offices with the rest of the group. From the outside, the building has very traditional, imposing stonework, but walking through the grand main entrance, we found ourselves in a vast modern atrium — a communal meeting area — of chrome and glass, stretching upwards, with each level of the building looking down on us.

We were treated to a presentation and discussion from Michael Barber, the prime minister's chief advisor on delivery. He encouraged us to be clear about our non-negotiables when setting key priorities, so as to remain accountable, but not so much as to compromise what was most important to us by too much. The phrase "dare to soar" was much discussed and another that I have often used since, "your attitude determines your altitude", and these phrases have continued to spur me on, despite any apparent setbacks or "arsonists" trying to undermine your work. As Paul was giving us all a tour around the building, we found ourselves standing outside the chancellor Gordon Brown's large imposing office door. We were like a group of wide-eyed children, knowing that the great man was actually in there at his desk and we were very conscious not to make lots of noise. However, we were soon greeted with a cheery "hello!"

from his special advisor, Ed Balls, hurrying by, looking quite bemused by us all, no doubt off to another important meeting. We spent more time during the rest of the day getting to know each other more, what our career and personal drivers were and how we had evolved as leaders in our fields. It was a very liberating and empowering experience which we reflected on together for a long time afterwards.

We regularly fed back to each other about what we had observed on each of our journeys. In writing this book, I took the opportunity of looking back at my notebook from the time and saw that AIG colleagues described me as: "softly spoken but very resilient; quietly ambitious; keeps to task to achieve outcomes". I have always believed that being a dietitian is no barrier to new challenges or opportunities, no matter how far removed they appear to be from the expected norm of those who cannot see outside the box. Thinking back over my career, I can recall several senior colleagues who have tried to pigeonhole me or limit my scope of practice, but, with my strong sense of self belief and a large pinch of determination, I have always persevered and overcome.

Our group went on to visit Killingbeck Police Station in Leeds one afternoon, where we were pleased to hear from a female chief inspector about the reality of working on the front line of the force. She described how officers were in charge in terms of their enforcement roles but we wondered how on earth could they possibly demonstrate transformational leadership in the ways that they worked? National targets on crime rates, numbers of arrests, crime prevention work, etc., surely ruled their lives. She described how the opportunity for transformation came down to senior officers at local level where the operational teams could discuss and decide on the best approach for their area. We discussed some flexibilities of developing their priorities and involvement in community projects, so another common stereotype had been dismissed. She went on to describe how training for junior officers promoted the "KISS" approach to police work — keep it simple, silly! We reflected that the most successful ideas are the simplest but people will still try to over-complicate initiatives, which often results in failure as you lose peoples' interest and struggle to engage them with your vision; it's true in every area of public life. Leadership is very much about not being afraid to admit that you've made a mistake or that you don't know something and it was empowering to hear the lived-out insights from a senior police officer, creating lots of discussion amongst our team. There will always be critics of your work, looking for any sign of failure or not quite hitting targets – the arsonists — but they are usually only hiding their own failings or inadequacies, happy to gaslight others to take the spotlight off their own lack of innovation and leader-ship qualities. I've seen and experienced so much of this kind of behaviour over the years, and I feel sorry for them. They rarely succeed in anything and others around notice their behaviour, which generally stifles creativity and generates fear and unhappiness in their teams. I often wonder what their personal or formative lives have been like to make them behave this way.

The chief inspector reflected on her experience of working with so many young people who turn to crime and what they had endured through their difficult upbringings, punctuated with lack of support, levels of violence or abuse towards them and a consequent lack of self-esteem. There were strong parallels with my conversations and experiences of working with so many of our young offenders, stuck in the revolving door life of prison.

Another day and another AIG experience, and I emerged from a tube station into the sunshine early one morning in 2004, clutching some instructions for directions to our next venue. It reminded me of a plot from a spy novel because I had been told to leave through a particular exit, walk across a narrow lane to an innocuous wooden door, set into a fairly unremarkable stone wall, and ring the buzzer outside. There were no details on the door to give any clue about what I might find inside; not even a number. Hearing a whirring sound, I looked up to see a CCTV camera focusing on me standing there. Just then, the door clicked open and I walked inside, just as my paper instructions had directed me to do. It was quite an astonishing entrance foyer. A long, winding chrome pathway — not unlike the airport security area — led me slowly down into the building and down towards a glass-fronted security desk. I presented my ID before being checked in and was escorted up several floors to meet with the others. Security was so tight that we weren't even allowed to go to the loo without an official escort, who would then stand outside and wait to take us back to the meeting room. To this day, I still have no idea what happened in the building but it was another of those unique experiences that the PSLS allowed us to access. It showed the level of trust that the cabinet office had in us and made us feel very special, which increased our "can do" attitude by letting us see that all things were possible. It was a powerful, almost addictive combination and we all thrived on it. My confidence and self-esteem continued to grow as I realised that personal self-belief wasn't confined to me and that others also appreciated my personality, skills and experiences.

Back in my day job, and as a member of the Medway PCT PEC and Board, I was equally supported by my chair and chief executive, Eddie and Bill, who encouraged me to take any opportunities for further development as they arose. It makes such a difference to be given the trust and the freedom to fly and it made it all the easier for me to start organising my interchange placement at national level. I started to work one day a week on secondment alongside the DH prison health team in Wellington House. By happy co-incidence, that brought me into contact with many more civil service colleagues and national agencies, which offered more career development possibilities and played a big part in my application for my next role. I also had access to more prisons around London, opening my eyes to more unique surroundings, the challenges of supporting inmates to stay well and to highlight opportunities to influence and recommend improved opportunities for a higher standard of nutritional care. I was delighted to be invited, with our department head, to visit the HMPS Director General, Phil Wheatley, in his office and was able to thank him once again for presenting me with my award for outstanding effort in prison healthcare. It was another "pinch me" moment as I would never have had that opportunity otherwise.

I was able to continue to work with the team until the middle of 2006 and Janet Waters arranged for me to be allocated a mentor who was based in Richmond House (the central locus of the Department of Health). I was quite amazed to meet him in his office — a large, well-furnished space — which looked directly onto Whitehall; a prime spot for anyone. He was encouraging and offered advice about maintaining integrity even when challenged by others' competing priorities and disruptive behaviours. The role of a civil servant seemed to me to be a complex game of chess, calm in the face of others' challenging manoeuvres and reliant on a network of supporting allies to succeed in whatever policy is being developed or delivered. I was sorry when he was promoted and moved away in yet another reshuffle, but his integrity in doing the right thing stayed with me. Whenever I walk down Whitehall, I look up at the window with fond memories, wondering who is based there now.

Chapter 10 — Volunteering with the BDA

During 39 years of membership (student and prac-tising), I was committed to continuously volunteering and was fortunate to have been elected to a variety of roles for the BDA. I've always felt proud to be a dietitian and consider it a real honour to have been able to play an active part in developing a strong profession for the future. I have seen firsthand the expansion and commitment to the continuous devel-opment of the association, the gradual growth of membership and numbers of employees and the relo-cations of premises, with several upgrades to larger, better-equipped offices across central Birmingham. I started my journey with the BDA as an industrial relations (IR) representative in 1987, during my first post in Sheffield, and I have always really enjoyed the opportunities to improve my general knowledge of the local and national NHS political strategies. After all, they have the potential to influence changes of working terms and conditions for fellow employees. I am a natural networker, curious to learn more about others' perspectives and experiences. Volunteering with the BDA also provided a great way of understanding and engaging with a variety of other organisations and their staff. There's no way that I'd have had those insights and opportunities just working in a local health board and, as someone once said to me, "You've got to be inside the tent to make change rather than being a bystander outside". In the days before the internet and instant electronic communication, my role as an IR steward offered me the quickest way of finding out firsthand about any health news or up to date information. Even though I was only a senior dietitian, this meant that I was able to be as up to date as local NHS senior managers and stewards from other unions. It was my job to consult with and share information with our members so that I could represent their views, concerns and insights to both the BDA and local management. At

JSCC meetings, the BDA was treated on a par with the much larger NUPE, NALGO and COHSE unions who were well-supported by national officers and full-time officials. At the time, the BDA had neither and I also represented views from the physiotherapists (CSP) and OTs (BAOT) which exposed me to a much better shared understanding of the broader AHP politics and issues.

In the late 1980s, there was a lot of co-ordinated industrial action, as unions proactively raised concerns about NHS pay and conditions. This led to a number of us heading down to London, one Saturday morning on a double decker bus, for a huge public sector protest march through the streets of the capital. All the way down the M1, fellow travellers tooted at us in support as we waved our banners from the windows and we felt quite exhilarated to be part of such an important national event. We proudly walked through the streets with the other health service unions, shouting key messages from megaphones and carrying huge banners, before joining together for a large rally and some rousing keynote speeches in Hyde Park. It all seemed to be going so well but my sense of exhilara-tion soon dropped as I felt a cold wet feeling on my leg, and despairingly, I realised that a carton of squash had leaked inside my jacket creating a large damp patch down the side of my trousers... I steamed all the way home to Sheffield in the back of the bus but it was all worth it in the end as pay scales finally started to increase a few months later.

I was desperately trying to get my first foothold on the booming housing ladder of the eighties and can remember calling my building society to arrange a bigger loan to cover my first-ever mortgage, when I discovered that my basic grade annual salary would be rising to just over £10,000. Up till then, I had been renting a room in the homes of colleagues and longed for more independence, while spending money on my own property rather than paying rent for someone else's. So, in 1988, at the age of 24, I became the proud owner of a 3-bedroom, classic Victorian mid- terraced home in the west end of the city, for the princely sum of £28,750. It was a great time of prosperity in prop-erty markets, and two years later, I sold it on for fifty percent more! Moving around the country throughout my career has also meant that I benefitted greatly from the previously generous workplace relocation costs and allowances, taking some extra financial pressure off and allowing me to continue investing in larger, nicer properties. It is another reason for being ever thankful for my NHS employment.

In 1991, my role as a BDA steward evolved further as I was elected to the position of regional representative for Trent — the largest NHS region in England at the time. I co-ordinated training, networking and development for the local BDA stewards in each of the health districts and we became a positive, supportive force together. I fondly remember the great camaraderie between us all, including Sheridan Waldron (Leicestershire), Sue Kellie (Mansfield), Lynne Hogan (Chesterfield), Tracey (Doncaster), Cyd Harrison (Barnsley) , Anne Pridgeon (Lincolnshire) and a lovely young woman from Nottingham whose name escapes me — but she had the most incredible engagement ring of huge diamonds and blue sapphires! We responded (by phone, letter and landline) to national consultations and fed back ideas for stewards' training to BDA head office, generally making sure that Trent stood out as a force for good, proactively representing our local members and influencing change for the workforce. At a national level, the BDA had established a national IR committee and in 1992, I was really humbled and honoured to be invited to join it, representing Trent. I was quite overawed to be among the some of the "big names" of the day. Norma Lauder was the elected Whitley Council representative, articulating BDA views on the PTA (professional and technical "A") bargaining committee. This was the national equivalent of "staff side", made up of delegates from professional trade unions meeting with national NHS leaders to submit evidence of the need to improve pay and conditions at work. She also worked for several decades as the dietetic services manager in Doncaster but went on to become the chair of the full Whitley Council. There was a general sense that she was a force to be reckoned with at all levels; none of us were in any doubt that she was in charge… She had a very stern appearance with hair tied back severely in a tight bun and she wore black-rimmed spectacles perched on her nose, which made her look far older than she actually was. You soon knew if she disagreed with anything you said as she fixed you with a paralysing stare, lips pursed, ready to challenge. Years later, I was completely blown away when she arrived at a national BDA conference, having decided to completely transform her look. Initially, none of us recognised her as her hair flowed freely at shoulder length; she was wearing contact lenses instead of glasses; her make- up was applied well and she was dressed in lovely bright colours. It took years off her and she really enjoyed the compliments combined with all the shocked reactions from those of us who she'd caught off guard. I came to know her better and have great respect for her as we worked more closely together. We have continued to bump into each other at professional events and share any news, opinion and reminiscences. Sibi Ramharry was the BDA general secretary of the late 80s while John Grigg was the lynchpin of the BDA office, employed as the "secretary" (the position has since been renamed CEO) to the organisation. He was fond of comparing his role with that of "Sir Humphrey", who many will remember from the comedy series of the day "Yes Minister". He was the power behind government; the chief civil servant, wisely advising, challenging and steering the changing, often inexperienced, ranks of elected key players through Council meetings and other strategic platforms. We had many frank and open conversations, and, on one occasion, he described me as being "magisterial". My initials at the time were E.R. — what can I say?! However, we actually had a healthy respect for each other and got on well despite any occasional professional differences. Years later, while I was working down in Kent, I was asked to join a specially invited gathering for his retirement dinner at a private members' club in London. Norma Lauder escorted him round each table as he welcomed everyone and reminisced during the evening. He was a well-respected figure and is still fondly remembered by everyone who had associations with the BDA at the time.

My fellow regional stewards in the late eighties and early 90s included Judith Hendry — succeeded by Fiona Gray (now Clark) — representing Scotland, Donna Duncan from Wales and Ruth Wood-Martin, a sports dietitian from Northern Ireland. Our contingent gradually increased over the coming few years to include Sandra Church from East Anglia and Caroline Quilty from Merseyside. Huge envelopes of papers and reports for and from meetings were posted out to us each month and we arrived for our discussions laden down with reading matter, much of which ended up in the bin afterwards; long before recycling or emails.

In time, Council, with some prompting from John, decided that we needed to develop our trade union services on a par with our professional counterparts and funded our first-ever full-time officer. We appointed David Wood, who was already an experienced full-time official, with years of experience of negotiating, bargaining and representing non-NHS public sector workers. He took a lot of pressure off John and brought a more focused, high-profile approach to BDA industrial relations. Together, we gradually became more organised over time and when Sibi stepped down as general secretary, Lynne Elliott was elected to her role for a two-year term of office. When Norma decided to stand down from the committee, we had to vote at the 1994 AGM for her replacement. Back then, we regularly had several hundred people turning up to listen to reports and to vote on key motions, filling large conference rooms in the Midlands. Most AGMs were held in Birmingham on a Saturday but that didn't stop us gathering. There was always robust discussion about proposed changes to the BDA constitution and who we all wanted to vote for. I stood against Jan Dawson from the Northwest of England to try and become the Whitley council representative, which caused a seismic shock amongst Council members at the time and there were frantic calls from "the establishment" to bolster votes for Jan, the Council nominee. Unsurprisingly, she got more votes than me (not by many though) to become the BDA Whitley Council representative and I continued to represent Trent on the national IR committee. My approach to any disappointments like this has always been to dust myself down, re-group and carry on regardless, so that I could get on with doing a good job in whatever role I had at the time and wait for other opportunities to come my way. I just accepted that it wasn't the right time and knew from others that having stood against a Council nominee, I had already really shaken things up and it would become clear that another, better role was waiting for me the following year.

The work of the trade union became busier, and we were soon able to appoint Nicky as a deputy for David, and Barbara as his secretary. We started organising regional stewards' training and development meetings. The first one was held over a weekend in Ironbridge, Shropshire, before later moving to a The Swallows Hotel in Solihull as a regular venue for several years to come. We invited speakers from fellow AHP trade unions and NHS managers like Neil MacKay from Sheffield, sharing best practice, developing and understanding our vision for the future of BDA as a trade union. In 1995, Lynne Elliott, our trade union general secretary, stood down after a two-year term in office and Council members nominated me to replace her. The AGM decision was decisive, and I was unanimously elected that summer, aged 31, making me the youngest-ever BDA trade union general secretary — what a huge honour. It was a very proud moment and meant stepping up to the heady altitude of the BDA Executive Committee, led by our Hon. Chairman Jane Eaton, Hon. Vice-chairman Sue Roberts, Hon. Treasurer Mary Cooper, Hon. Secretary Susan Jones of Sheffield, and the Hon. Education Officer the late Pat Judd, followed by Margaret Lawson, all the time ably supported by the BDA secretary John Grigg. We were the key decision-making committee for the profession, developing and taking strategic plans, vision and proposals to the larger BDA Council meetings, which met each quarter. A huge A4 envelope of papers would thud on the doormat the week before, carefully prepared by John and the very small office team at the time. There were lots of telephone and face-to-face conversations, but a great deal of effort, not to mention travel between Manchester and Birmingham, was needed to keep up with the Council sub committees, BDA business and representation on behalf of members. Mobile phones were still in their infancy and IT infrastructure — never mind the world wide web — was negligible.

BDA conferences of the early to mid-90s were huge events, running over three days at a large conference centre in Stratford upon Avon. It was quite normal to have more than 400 paying participants each day, with staff of all grades coming from every corner of the UK to be part of the event. The Scientific Programmes Committee was chaired at the time by Susan Jones, with enthusiastic support from Anne Robinson, Michelle Rae, Sue Kellie, Jill Ward and Luci Daniels. They were responsible for delivering it all, which meant extensive, very detailed planning and organisation, but they never disappointed. The conferences attracted big name keynote scientific and professional speakers, who delivered presentations on the nutritional science and research of the day. There were huge volumes of industry sponsorship taking up several large exhibition halls full of stands overflowing with information, emerging products, merchandise and competitions. Conference dinners usually included something entertaining too. We had a medieval dinner at Warwick Castle (not everyone enjoyed the experience of having to eat with their fingers, though); Pam Ayres was a very amusing after-dinner speaker one year; line dancing was quite hilarious at another event; and a big industry partner even sponsored a boat trip and dinner down the Avon. It was one of the very few disasters of the conference seasons because by the time we had all climbed aboard our barge and set off, the sun rapidly went down, leaving us all crowded inside — no nice summer scenery — eating pub food for a couple of hours below deck, with the pungent aroma of engine fuel and smoke, desperate to get off again. Despite that, there was regularly great support from the member-ship for national and local events, which continued to grow, resulting in lots of dietitians becoming keen to volunteer to be part of various committees needed for the work of the Association. At the 1995 event, I was stunned to discover that my name had been randomly selected out of a hat for a prize draw organised by one of the company stands. Unbelievably, I had won a state-of-the-art food processor. I was stunned, surprised and anxious all at the same time as memories of my catering practical sessions at RGU came rushing through my mind, thinking of the disastrous efforts at making egg mayonnaise a decade previously! In a weird, ironic twist of co-incidence, my lecturer from back then, Janet Lowell, was at the conference in her new role as a nutritional advisor to a large, multinational confectionery company and afterwards, we had a bit of a laugh about my win.

In due course, members of the BDA council decided that we should hold our first smaller conference in Glasgow although there were still around three hundred participants at the packed event. As we sat down for the conference dinner, it was announced that Carole Middleton (from my days in Leeds), sitting at a neighbouring table, had become the first dietitian to be awarded an MBE for her work in the world of sports nutrition. We all applauded and congratulated her, sharing the joy and pride as a professional body. Since then, several more of my colleagues have also received honours from the late Queen, who was, co-incidentally, the patron of the BDA.

It had been agreed that the trade union would have a full afternoon, promoting and sharing issues related to members' concerns in an open discussion and it took the form of a Q&A with David ready to answer questions from the floor. There was a huge turnout – about 200 people had stayed for the session — and it went far better than any of us could have expected, with dietitians from all over the UK joining in.

There were no devolved governments or differing health strategies at that time, so there were lots of common issues, policies and concerns about NHS terms and conditions of service from across the UK-wide profession. It's often said that we are a very small AHP organisation, where everyone knows who everyone else is and it was so true that afternoon. I was able to introduce every single person who asked him a question. I doubt very much that I'd be able to do that today as the membership is so much larger and more diverse with fewer opportunities now for us all to meet in such large numbers. Sadly today, AGMs and BDA conferences attract far less interest or partic-ipation and company sponsorship has dwindled to a few core businesses. Industry sponsors now include large multi-nationals, which has caused lots of debate and dissatisfaction amongst many of the membership, but it is a feature of the world of business that the BDA operates in today. Voting for proposals at AGMs rarely gets close to a hundred votes; a fraction of the thousands of members who could potentially have a say. It's hard to know the reason for that but possibly a mix of lack of funding from NHS employers, busy workloads and challenging financial times for conventional sponsors. It's disappointing for those of us who can remember the heydays of Stratford where members enjoyed meeting up and networking with colleagues, embracing more personal connections and taking joint responsibility for BDA business.

I temporarily re-joined the BDA Council from 2007-8 as the deputy Scottish constituency council member, supporting Helen Davidson in her role as Board chair. However, workforce challenges in the dietetic team at work back then meant that I had to step back and focus all my time on the day job. Staffing numbers had increased, with new investment complicated by various periods of maternity leave, which took time to recruit for. Organisational restructuring combined with the general challenges of dietetic service management also meant that I would have to bide my time and wait before re-focusing on a volunteering role for the BDA again.

The opportunity came again in 2013 when I was co-opted to join the BDA Council, primarily for two years from 2014-2016. This time, I became the deputy Scottish constituency representative supporting the BDA Scotland board chair, Marjory MacLeod. We both had a place on the national BDA Council, representing the interests of the profession in Scotland. There was a good mix of specialist members on our committee — freelance, industry, public health, social care and learning difficulties — from all over the country. We were always looking for ways to raise the profile of dietitians and contribute to the development of health policy and standards of care. I represented the BDA, along with other AHPs, at political party events and helped develop an event at the Scottish parliament. It focused on the important role of dieti-tians across Scotland in supporting people living with dementia. It tied in well with the work being done by Prof Elaine Hunter at Alzheimer Scotland and was well received. I suggested that we could consider starting to plan a national conference, specifically for Scottish dietitians, to showcase best practice, and celebrate the BDA's upcoming 80th anniversary in September 2016. I was asked by Marjory and the rest of the team to take on the role of organising it and I began by chairing a working group to turn the idea into action. I was grateful to have support from a proactive group of colleagues representing a variety of areas, including RGU, NES, Industry, the BDA, SDLN and the two Scottish BDA branches. By now, Tracy MacInnes had taken on the role of interim Chief Health Professions Officer for the Scottish government. Her team of senior AHP leaders all got behind us and we secured a top-notch selection of speakers, 3rd sector partners and industry exhibitors, all of which helped to make sure the event, at The Carnegie conference centre in Dunfermline, became a sell-out. The BDA Chairman, Fiona McCulloch, opened the day in front of a capacity audience and congratulated us on all our efforts. We had a mixture of keynote speakers, workshops and poster presentations, which attracted a great range of entries from most Boards. Prizes were donated from a variety of organisations, and it was great to have colleagues from all but a couple of small health boards actively contributing. There was a huge buzz in the venue as people caught up with each other, reminiscing, sharing and celebrating the day. I was really pleased to see two of my former RGU peers, Lindsay and Spike (of the moleskin coat) and we had a short time to update each other about our lives and the others from our course before I was pulled back into conference activities. The exhibition stands weren't quite on the scale of the famous Stratford conferences of the 90s but there was a great variety from the enteral feeding industry, leaving little space for anyone else. We also had third sector colleagues from Alzheimer Scotland and the Food Standards Agency. Staff from the BDA work-ready programme and trade union also added an extra dimension of learning and engagement. After a fantastic lunch, our celebration cake was cut by the BDA Chair to a round of clapping and cheering. It had been made by Alison, one of our committee members, who was co-incidentally also a professional cake-maker in her spare time. It had been the first-ever BDA conference for Scottish dietitians and as I stood up to close the event and present the much-anticipated poster prizes, I reflected that, as with all attempts to do things first and taking a very innovative approach to the event, we had experienced criticism, doubt and pessimism from some quarters. Innovation requires a degree of risk-taking but the profession in Scotland wanted an event of their own, so they had spoken up and, with a united effort, it had been success-fully delivered. I closed the conference, reflecting on my own career history, in and through my personal experiences of the previous 4 decades of BDA anni-versaries. I felt huge overwhelming pride, standing in front of so many colleagues, from students, up to senior members of the profession of the day. It was also great to have past Honorary Chairs, Edith Elliott and Helen Davidson, in the audience, letting others see that they should also aspire to high office in the BDA. The venue was unusually still packed at the end of the day, and we presented prizes for the top three posters, judged by the audience members throughout the event.

I was surprised but delighted to be presented with a lovely floral bouquet by Janie Gordon, chair of the Scottish Dietetic Leadership group, announcing to the audience, "She's our leader!" and I headed back north on a career high. I hope that future Scottish dietitians will feel encouraged to build on the first event and to share their work, promoting the versatile role of the profession to the public, NHS, social care and voluntary sectors.

Soon after, I was invited to become a member of the BDA Investigation and Disciplinary Committee, which I continued to participate in up until retirement. It still meant travelling to and staying over in Birmingham for occasional meetings and it gave me the chance to keep in contact with the office staff, although there was also an annual opportunity to join a telephone Council conference call which was some respite. I enjoyed being back in the centre of BDA business planning, governance and oversight but also really loved working with members from other parts of the UK and hearing about what was happening in the wider profession. BDA offices had very little in the way of digital opportunities for members to join committees, which disadvantaged many from remote and rural areas, where return travel to Birmingham could take an unacceptable 2-3 days out of their working week. During the COVID pandemic of 2020, the BDA board of directors pragmatically and essentially decided to transform ways of working, making far better use of new technologies and platforms to engage with members. It helped in maintaining the business of the association and ensured that the BDA public profile remained high. This was enthusiastically welcomed by the profession and our partners as it allowed support for core business and committee meetings, webinars and members' training events, for the recruitment and appointment process for a new board of directors and it also drastically reduced costs of travel time and associated subsistence claims.

Chapter 11 — Affiliation with the TUC

The IR Committee of the 1990s included six regional stewards from across the UK, a Whitley council representative, David the full-time officer and me as general secretary in the chair. We had responsibility for preparing reports for Council members, while developing and sharing our strategic vision to raise the profile and influence of the BDA on national public sector issues. David and I regularly met with other PAM trade union officials from the Chartered Society of Physiotherapists (CSP), British Orthoptic Society (BOS) and Society of Radiographers (SOR) in their various headquarters, which were all within walking distance of Euston Station in London. Many of our contemporaries were already developing stronger partnerships with the TUC, raising the profile and issues of their membership to highlight their contribution to the healthcare sector. It was in this context that in the autumn of 1996, at the end of a two-day meeting of regional stewards in Solihull, we met with John Monks, TUC general secretary of the time, to consider a step up into the high-profile world of the well-oiled and highly co-ordinated left-wing political machine. He arrived in his chauffeur-driven Jaguar and chatted very genially with us, stressing the many benefits to a small organisation like ours. We, in turn, reflected that we would potentially bring some more balance and credibility from the BDA, mainly female membership. This was in direct contrast to the traditional view of the TUC representing many of the hard left, male-dominated, traditional busi-nesses which employed so many manual workers. We took our recommendation to join up back to the BDA executive committee then on to the wider National Council before seeking approval from all members at the AGM. Thankfully, the majority agreed with us and the proposal was carried; our plan to become affili-ated to the TUC began in earnest. At the time, I was working in Oldham, in the NW of England, and was invited, with David, to represent the Association as observers at the 1996 TUC congress, which was held that year in Blackpool. It was around the time that the BDA office staff had joined the GMB and David took great pleasure in introducing me to their larger than life general secretary, John Edmonds, as "The BDA management!" I had a bit of an "imposter syndrome" moment and felt so lucky to observe all the big union names of the time at close quarters: Bill Morris of the huge Transport and General Workers' Union; Arthur Scargill from the NUM and representatives from the powerful Iron and Steel Workers' Trades Confederation. Bob Abberley was the head of UNISON, Phil Gray from the CSP then the RCN, and I was relieved to see counterparts from some of the other national PAMs organisations.

Within the year, we became fully affiliated to the TUC and the BDA's IR committee soon decided it was time that we stepped up as TUC members and present our inaugural motion to the next conference in Brighton. It took some time to decide which topic we would speak about but eventually, we concluded that it needed to shine the spotlight on the management of malnutrition — a theme which sadly still continues to cause concern today. As the trade union general secretary, I had the task of preparing and presenting our motion for congress members to vote on. This created some tension with BDA PENG (parenteral and enteral nutrition group) members but after some behind-the-scenes discussions, we reached a cordial agreement. The main factor was that the issue was raised, and it didn't matter that it was a trade unionist delivering it — I was a dietitian after all. I was so glad to have the support of both my manager and the rest of my dietetic team, who had to cover my clinic work while I was away for most of the week. Originally, I was due to speak on day 3, so had plenty of opportunity to see how things worked, to network and prepare myself for my inaugural speech, which should have been streamed live on national TV. When the big day arrived, David and I found ourselves in the front row seats designated for new affiliates and speakers. However, it soon became clear that this was going to be no ordinary day when David was asked whether we would mind delaying our slot, due just before lunchtime, to allow a surprise speaker to address congress. At midday, Tony Blair, the newly elected Labour prime minister, stepped forward into the centre of the stage and into my presentation slot… There was rapturous applause from every corner of the conference floor where the atmosphere was highly charged. It was a really memorable occasion for David and me, as we looked on to the unfolding scene from the luxury of our front-row seats! There was a huge feeling of euphoria and expectation after years of disputes with central government and I'm sure that the Prime Minister went home with applause ringing in his ears. I didn't know it at the time but my lovely granny, a lifelong Labour voter, was sitting at home in the north of Scotland, glued to the TV, waiting for my speech and wondering why he was there instead, but I would have to wait another two days before being given the opportunity to finally deliver our motion to the gathered masses. I was thankful to see that by then, the national TV press had dismantled their camera equipment and left for the weekend. As I walked forward and stepped onto the stage, the vast size of the audience in the Brighton conference centre struck me full force and I steadied myself, aware that David was poised below the podium with the BDA camera, ready to capture some history for the association. I started by introducing myself from the BDA — "a new affiliate". There was a traditional round of loud, welcoming clapping and cheering as congress members do for all first-timers. It took my breath away a bit but I carried on with my well-rehearsed speech, keeping one eye on the traffic light timer to my right which I had been told would gradually change colour from green to red when I reached the end of my allotted slot. I managed to maintain my composure when the amber light flashed, finishing my motion before sitting back down with loud applause all around from all the delegates and beaming congratulations from David. I looked up to the podium and was greeted with a friendly, encouraging thumbs up from Brendan Barber, John Monks' deputy, who would go on to become the TUC general secretary himself several years later. We were delighted to report back to Council that our first BDA motion had been unanimously supported by the Congress representatives. BDA trade union staff and represent-atives have continued to raise issues that are important to members at a far wider range of TUC events both nationally and within the home countries. I still feel very proud of my part in forming and contributing to the association's successful longstanding partnership with our trade union colleagues.

By the AGM of 1998, I had been elected to the posi-tion of BDA Hon. Vice-chairman, supporting our new Hon. Chairman, Alison Dobson, a fellow Scot who was well liked and worked with a quiet, determined way. We were all very shocked and sad when she was diagnosed with cancer and passed away a couple of years later. She was one of many BDA chairs that I have served with over my career, including: Loretta Cox, Luci Daniels, Susan Jones, Sue Roberts, Judith Catherwood, Helen Blackwell, Fiona McCulloch and Sian O'Shea. My time as BDA Vice-Chair was short-lived though, as I discovered early on that I was now pregnant… with twins. Had I only had one baby to care for, I might have taken him/her with me to BDA meetings, just as Sue Roberts had managed to do with her son James several years earlier. As it turned out, I was advised by medical staff to start my maternity leave in early winter, so I stepped back from both my substantive role in Oldham and my BDA duties in November 1998. I rented my house to Karen, one of our dietitians, and temporarily returned to my hometown in Scotland, where my daughters were safely delivered by planned C-section in January 1999. It was more than a year later before I could return to any kind of active participation in any BDA voluntary work but John and some of the office staff and Council colleagues kept in touch during my time away, which was a nice way to stay connected.

When I moved to work in Kent in July 1999, David and John asked me to use my past experience to support several areas of work, including a dietetic service review in a neighbouring health board, assessing the clinical practice of a registrant, and working with David and the regional stewards to consider and discuss the implementation of the new Agenda For Change (A4C) pay scales and the implementation of the Knowledge and Skills Framework (KSF). For practical reasons, juggling a busy job and bringing up twin toddlers, I didn't have the time or the energy to take up any formal BDA voluntary positions but I continued to keep in touch with David and the office staff. On a few occasions, they also passed my name to health boards that were looking for an independent expert for dietetic management interview panels or service reviews. I mainly travelled around the NHS in the Southeast of England but had the chance to fly over to Ireland in 2001, at the request of local dietetic management, so that I could spend a few days shadowing a registrant and providing an independent professional view about her ability to practice safely. I flew into Belfast airport late one afternoon and had a bit of a starstruck moment as a small group of men walked past me. I looked out the corner of my eye and clearly recognised the familiar face of George Best… Then, having walked past him, I turned round for a final look just as he did the same at me — probably wondering what I was doing. In quite a surreal moment, we gave a nonchalant nod towards each other and carried on with our business.

The dietitian concerned was thankfully very open to my presence beside her in clinic settings and was able to reflect on her practice with me afterwards. Sadly, it became very clear quite quickly that her knowledge of clinical dietetics was not as one might have expected. I distinctly remember her telling a patient, newly diagnosed with insulin dependent diabetes, that the best thing he could do was eat "pure and gentle foods". She repeated this several times in the course of the conversation and the poor man left with a diet sheet and a very confused expression. I made sure afterwards that he was contacted separately by one of the other members of the department to provide more evidence-based advice and support. My report, detailing several concerns and failings, was shared with the dietetic services manager and the case went to a CPSM hearing. I was invited to their main offices in Kennington Road to provide evidence at the hearing related to considering her ability to practice. She didn't attend or attempt to offer any defence herself and was subsequently struck off the register as the evidence of unsafe practice — mine included— was overwhelming. Fortunately, such cases against dietitians are very rare. Several years previously, as general secretary of the trade union, I had been invited to Kennington Road to observe a hearing against a young member who had been referred by her employer for various aspects of poor record-keeping. The BDA, in the form of David, on behalf of the national IR committee, supported her case and had arranged a variety of supportive witnesses in her defence. I went on to write an article for the members' magazine expressing my concern that she had had so little support from her employer to improve her practice. I felt that it was important for the membership to recognise that more dietitians were sadly being referred to the CPSM for reasons of poor record-keeping. The BDA Professional Development Committee, with input from David and the Industrial Relations Committee, went on to work jointly with the CPSM to develop a common set of record-keeping standards, which continue to provide clear and equitable guidance for members. Referrals to the regulator significantly reduced, and even today, there are very few examples of dietitians being specifically referred for concerns about this area of practice.

In the early 2000s, while I was based in Kent, work to revolutionise the NHS pay structure saw the introduction of the Knowledge and Skills Framework (KSF). I was invited by David Wood to join a meeting of regional stewards to help explain how these would work in practice and the implications for successfully engaging members in implementing the new Agenda For Change pay scales. Unbeknown to me, Carolyn Bell, one of my RGU contemporaries, was also there as she was now a regional steward in the East of England; the first of many future encounters with colleagues from Aberdeen days. Dietetics continues to be a very small world! It was good to take time to hear about the classmates that she continued to keep in contact with; Caroline, Lindsay and Wendy. Little did I know that I would meet Lindsay back in Scotland more than 15 years later.

The career structure for dietitians was still quite limited, with very few support worker roles, apart from limited secretarial help, often shared with other teams. Members working in clinical specialities often found themselves stuck at the top of a pay scale with limited opportunity to progress financially or professionally, unless they moved from a clinical role into management. There was a commonly held view in some areas that there was no point employing basic grade dietitians in specialist areas, citing a (short-sighted) view that they lacked experience and skill. However, over time, and with further investment in specialist services, teams developed with a broader range of all grades – initially in tertiary paediatric units like Great Ormond Street. There was also an expectation that if you started your career specialising in one clinical area, you were then committed to doing that forever. I consider myself to have been very fortunate to have been able to move job roles over the years across several areas of practice — burns/plastics, renal, ITU, prisons, sport, freelance and social care.

Student training was an optional role for dietetic teams and it came with an additional 3-tiered financial allowance. Dietitians refused to take students without being paid this, and sadly, not all employers were willing to fund it. Many highly specialist teams refused to have students on placement, taking the view that they would be training staff to become basic grades but wouldn't then be able to employ them. It was a short-term view because, at some point in the future, those basic grades might have chosen to apply for senior specialist roles with them. Most student placements were centred in acute teams, which was still where the majority of the profession practised. There were pockets of part-time community dietitians but many senior colleagues generally felt that they would never be able to manage to sustain a student placement programme. The trend was broken by a consortium of community dietitians in the southwest of England who demonstrated that students could have a productive, enjoyable placement experience in different locations if they were supervised by a number of part-time colleagues. All it took was good plan-ning and a well-coordinated timetable and excellent communication between all parties. Over the years, we have gradually seen an increase in the range of student placements in a greater variety of settings and specialities, including the army, the food industry, the media, social care and even the BDA offices. There are no longer separate training allowances as the Agenda For Change pay system reflected them in pay scales and there is an expectation that all members of NHS dietetic teams now offer and support training opportunities. We moved on to a more radical system of student training ten years later, in response to a noticeable reduction in dietitians completing their practical placements. Often, many of them dropped out in their final year, having been put off by being exposed to the harsh reality and challenges of a hospital environment, coming face-to-face with the sight of seriously ill patients. It was decided that exposure to clinical environments early in their training would give them the chance to decide that if they didn't like it, they could transfer to another non-clinical course without wasting four years of study. And so the A, B, C system developed, allowing even more dietetic teams to support placements. There is still a view, particularly in some acute settings, that students should only be trained in hospital environments. However, as a profession, it is critical that we take a longer-term view and consider how to develop and promote the core skills and professional qualities that we'll need to support the health service of the future.

There will be a more diverse community health and social care infrastructure where dietitians will be central to transforming traditional models of supporting good health and well-being. Who would have thought, when I trained back in the 80s, alongside 2nd year pharmacy students, that dietitians would one day go on to become trained prescribers? The possibilities are endless if we open our minds to release the potential we have in our core skill sets, supporting, encouraging and celebrating the possibilities of innovation.

Chapter 12 — A national role

In the autumn of 2005, I became aware of a fantastic new and previously unforeseen career opportunity. The National Patient Safety Agency (NPSA), one of the Department of Health's "arm's length bodies" of the day, advertised a newly created post. I thought the job description could have been written for me— Head of Nutrition and Cleaning for England and Wales. I would be working with a diverse team developing best practice for pharmacy, human factors and a range of safer practice initiatives. The focus of my role was to identify areas, related to nutrition and cleaning, which might be putting patients at risk of harm. My small team then had to develop national advice or guidance notices, to mitigate against it happening across the NHS. Our partners in both Scotland and Northern Ireland invariably adopted these as well. I was interviewed at NPSA headquarters on a morning of torrential rain and made it from the nearby tube station to the building in plenty of time but looking quite damp and dishevelled! Fortunately, the lovely receptionist took pity on me and offered to hang up my saturated brolly and wet coat. I managed to sort out my hair and make-up, gathering myself together while all the time wondering who else I might be up against. I didn't have long to wait to find out when someone I knew from my time working in Trent region emerged, giving me a sheepish smile as she quickly headed out into the storm. I was interviewed by my (soon-to-be) new manager, Dr Helen Glenister, along with Liz Jones from the DH Estates team in Leeds, which had previously hosted the cleaning and patient engagement elements of the role. I had a tight remit to deliver a presentation within a strict time limit, while all the time trying to make a strong impression. We then moved onto the questions and I found myself able to offer a range of examples from my leadership roles, as PEC Chair, at NOMS and on the cabinet office leadership scheme. Liz was keen to explore my understanding of the challenges for NHS domestic staff. Somehow, from the depths of my memory, I managed to pull some relevant examples and insights from my work as a hospital domestic during university holidays in Aberdeen. We were all still smiling when I left the interview and I headed back out to the reception area, anticipating the dampness of my coat and the wet weather outside again. Chatting away to the receptionist, I spotted another well-known "competitor" trying unsuccessfully to sit out of my line of vision. We nodded knowingly at each other and I left him to it. Heading back to Kent on the train a couple of hours later, I was delighted to receive the phone call I'd been waiting for from Helen and I grinned like a Cheshire cat all the way home. I called my "mentor," Mary at NOMS, who was thrilled to hear my news and we arranged to celebrate when I was next at Wellington House.

While I worked my notice in Kent, I was able to participate in the interviews for one of the posts, which would sit below me at the NPSA — the head of nutrition. There was a strong field of candidates from a variety of settings and I joined Helen to interview three of them at the NPSA offices in December 2005. We were able to easily offer the post to Caroline Lecko who had been doing some fantastic work to improve nutritional care, while working as an NHS modern matron in a large London teaching hospital. She demonstrated great organisational skills, a proactive approach and clear commitment to ensuring that high-quality care was delivered safely to patients. Colleagues from dietetics, the PEC and Board members gave me several lovely send-offs; more flowers than I had vases for and lots of generous gifts, before I started my new role in January 2006.

Getting to work started at 6 am, by catching a commuter coach to Canary Wharf from my home in Sittingbourne, before changing to the underground on the Jubilee then Victoria lines. It was a daily four-hour commute and most of the journey was in darkness so I saw very little, which made it quite monotonous. I have no idea how so many manage to maintain this sort of lifestyle for years at a time and I have since reflected that the quality of many people's lives must have been vastly improved during the COVID lockdown when they were released from the tortures of the daily grinding commute to work on crowded trains and buses. Arriving for my first week, I was warmly welcomed to the patient safety team and started a round of induction meetings getting to know everyone and making connections with other teams. I soon realised that I already had lots of helpful links from other government departments, which I had developed during my time working at Wellington House and with colleagues on the Cabinet Office's public sector leadership scheme. It certainly made it easier for me to have conversations with the Chief Nursing Officer's (CNO) team at Richmond House, notably Kay East, the Chief Allied Health Professions Officer at the time, who I had first met at a meeting of Southeast England dietetic managers. She had been surprised and delighted to hear that I was the deputy chair of a PEC and promoted my work even more when I was appointed as the first-ever dietetic PEC chair. Her office in the basement of Wellington House was just a few floors below the NOMS team and she actively encouraged me to pop down for a coffee and chat whenever I was in the building. She was incredibly approachable and clearly very keen to hear about the role AHPs were playing in lots of different settings and she struck me as a very person-centred caring individual, keeping patients at the centre of conversations. At one national AHP event, she introduced me to the CNO, Christine Beasley, and I was able to remind her that she had presented me with a Kent regional health authority "Inequalities in Health Award" back in 2002 for my innovative work with prisoners. She had a very friendly but professional manner and was a great role model for health service leadership, focused on the front line service and the care of patients. Our paths crossed on various committees during my time at the NPSA and Kaye enabled me to have easy access to share and inform the national team about the projects my team were working on. Helen and my peers on the patient safety team were surprised by this informal approach, as my contemporaries had to follow a much more formal route for engaging with their links at the Department of Health. Helen recognised that I had an ability to build strong, wide-ranging professional networks and that I was able to get things done differently, so she was more than happy to give me the autonomy of working using my unique approach. It was during my time at the NPSA that I first came across Project Initiation Documents (PIDs) and their management. They were generally referred to as "paralysing into despair" because of the tortuous level of detail needed and length of time taken to get them approved after navigating a strict unyielding internal approvals process. I had no formal training in project management and relied very much on others in the team and the wider agency to help me articulate the work we were trying to deliver. I am very self-aware and know my capabilities but the level of concentration and mind-numbing need to build a detailed, data-filled business case for each version was certainly not one of them! Other team leads were so much better at this and we all recognised each other's strengths. Mine was much more in developing and connecting colleagues from many cross-sector agencies and organisations, as diverse as central government and third-sector partners. I was pleased to be able to continue my work with the prison health team for one day a week for the first few months of the new role and found myself bumping into various people across Whitehall who had been on the PSLS programme. I also maintained a close, positive relationship with my own profession, including Judith Catherwood, the Hon. Chair of the BDA, and in time, we would go on to work together in the Highlands. It was a real honour for a me, as a dietitian, to have such a unique national role and people were curious to hear about and contribute to why nutrition and cleaning were patient safety issues. In the first fortnight of January, I joined Helen and the team in Birmingham for the prestigious National Patient Safety Conference. It was a huge event, bringing together high-profile international and UK speakers, exhibitors and participants spanning a wide range of sectors, covering an enormous range of topics. It was a quick and overwhelming immersion into my new work environment but at least I wasn't expected to deliver any speeches at it. Helen had already told me that I had been "booked" to present at several other national events in the coming months, so I was able to meet some of the main contacts who'd be introducing me as the keynote speaker at their various podiums. They included the Association of Domestic Managers (ADM), The Hospital Caterers' Association (HCA) and The British Dietetic Association (BDA), at their 70th anniversary celebrations. At the ADM event, I spoke for 20 minutes before being ushered to a chair on the stage where I faced a Q&A session led by a journalist who fielded questions from the audience. My briefings helped me through the event as I talked about our working priorities for the coming year, where aspects of research into hospital cleaning practices were being explored with partners at the DH and a large London University Hospital team. I was thankful to be able to finish and left the event feeling relatively unscathed -relieved to get some positive feedback from Helen when I got back at the office. I travelled north on the train late one afternoon in preparation for the HCA event, which was being held in a large Midlands hotel the next day. Stepping out of the international railway station, I spotted a waiting taxi and got into the back seat. The driver announced that he was already booked for a private client and as I was about to gather my things together ready for a hasty exit, a large man got into the front passenger seat. The driver said something to him and he turned round and, in a very deep Russian accent, offered to drop me off at my hotel. I was too tired to refuse so I happily accepted and we talked on the journey about each other's trips. He was apparently a banker, travelling for business between Moscow and the UK. We stopped to refuel at a service station before carrying on to the large hotel and conference centre where I thanked him for his generosity and headed inside. As I relayed my journey to Liz Jones (from the DH Estates team) the next day over coffee, her shocked expression made me realise that maybe I needed to consider my own safety a bit more before accepting lifts from strange Russian bankers (or any others) in future...

The next day, as I stood up to speak to the hundreds of HCA delegates, I introduced myself as having come from a background in prison health, which had quite a different take on safety compared to my new role. It broke the ice and helped me settle into my rehearsed presentation, which was thankfully well received. I'm not sure how I managed to stay calm, having been briefed about a new policy just seconds before stepping up to the microphone. I just hoped that no one would ask me a question related to it at the Q&A session afterwards.

Working in central London, I was regularly back and forwards to Richmond House for committee meetings with the CNO or members of her team. On one occasion, Helen and I were asked to meet with the latest junior health minister to describe our planned approach to the nutrition and cleaning agenda. We arrived at the minister's office and were ushered into a waiting room, having been told that we would be admitted for the meeting once we had been joined by another participant. A short while later, the door opened and in walked Lloyd Grossman, the larger-than-life face of the "better hospital food" programme and lead for the development of a national menu for English hospitals. He and Helen had clearly met previously and the conversation was very informal and genial. We were ushered through to meet the female minister and, after a short chat, Lloyd and I headed down in the lift together. He shouted his hellos to a couple of other government ministers as the doors opened at various floors below and we went our separate ways onto Whitehall but never had the opportunity to meet again. One of my other roles, which came with the job, was to have the overall NHS lead for the annual PEAT (Patient Environment and Action Team) survey across hospital sites in England and Wales. It was a function that used to sit with the NHS Estates team, focusing on non-clinical services, and we were fortunate to have Gemma to continue keeping us on track with her skills and expertise. The public are generally happy to give their views about hospital experience — cleaning standards and general environmental factors such as paintwork, standard of food, and politeness of staff to name a few. Patient representatives joined small teams of evaluators, including facilities staff from neighbouring board areas to score all the factors in their local hospital sites. Once completed, and rated with the rest of England and Wales, the PEAT comparisons were published annually for national agencies to consider and build into their own strategic work plans. Helen tasked me with reviewing the value of PEAT, which involved consulting with all our national partners to establish how helpful the survey feedback was for their work streams and in planning future changes to delivery of services. It was really interesting to hear just how many other areas of the non-NHS agencies respected and relied on the feedback. I was able to conclude that the work was highly valued and that PEAT surveys should continue to be supported, which was then fed back to the NPSA Board. The conclusion from their discussions was very positive and the work was thankfully allowed to continue.

Throughout 2006, a personal drama was also unfolding in my life as my mother, living alone hundreds of miles away in the north of Scotland, was becoming much frailer, due to the effects of a cancer recurrence and spread. I found myself having to fly to Aberdeen several times during various acute hospital admissions and it gradually reached a point where I couldn't sustain a busy national career while balancing the needs of my family. In August, I took two weeks' annual leave as school holidays got underway and took the decision that I needed to plan a move back to my hometown in Scotland.

I confirmed that Helen was happy for me to change my working arrangements like others in the team and started the process of selling my house in Kent. The NPSA was very much ahead of many employers at the time, allowing me the opportunity of working from home in Scotland on Monday, travelling to London in the late evening to stay in a Euston hotel when working Tuesday to Thursday at NPSA headquarters before flying back north on Thursday evening and working from home on the Friday. It just wasn't a sustainable — or affordable — solution and, in the end, the situation came to a head in September forcing me to make a major life-changing decision. I knew that I had to put my family before work, no matter how successful my role at the NPSA was, and that I'd have to find a way of relocating to the north of Scotland.

In the monthly BDA vacancy bulletin, I noticed that a dietetic manager's post had been advertised in Inverness, so I made some tentative enquiries and arranged an informal coffee and chat about it with the professional lead, scheduled for the following Friday when I was home for the weekend. I took the pragmatic view that if I could at least get some permanent work in the Highlands, it would allow me to transition into the Scottish health service, take some financial pressure off and allow me to focus more time on my family priorities while I needed to. Having never worked in Scotland, I felt a bit uncomfortable about stepping across the border but felt that I would soon get to grips with the system. I discovered that there had been a vacancy for a manager in the Raigmore Hospital dietetic team for nearly a year. Previous recruitment attempts, including two rounds of unsuccessful interviews, had failed so I was hopeful that I might have a more positive experience. During September and October, I had a couple of further informal meetings, including a visit to the team office, before the professional head of service informed me that she would be happy for me to apply for the post. I realised that it would be a huge drop in salary and responsibility, but I was prepared to live with that in the interim just to have a regular income. I needed to find a way of supporting my family while continuing to practice as a dietitian. I had simultaneously been offered part-time work in Aberdeen but the distance and further reduced salary simply meant I had no choice but to decline. With a heavy heart, I took a leap of faith and gave Helen two months' notice. NPSA colleagues and those from partner agencies, including HMPS, were equally understanding, though disappointed at my decision. Kay East, the chief Health Professions Officer, contacted me directly to tell me how sorry she was to hear my news, as we had forged a very positive working relationship. She could see that I hadn't taken my decision lightly but encouraged me to focus on my family while I still could. I was relieved to be invited for interview in Inverness and prepared a PowerPoint presentation on how I hoped to develop the dietetic service for the future. It was scheduled for the last Friday in October — the day after my final day working in London; talk about cutting it fine! In the week leading up to it, I was so ill with a heavy cold and had been unable to travel to Leeds to deliver a presentation to a national caterers' event. Staying in a budget hotel near Earl's Court, I wondered how on earth I was going to have enough energy to get into the office next day to hand over my equipment and say my goodbyes before heading back to Aberdeen via Luton Airport. It was one of the worst journeys I've ever experienced as we flew north in an awful storm. The wind buffeted us everywhere and we nearly didn't manage to land as conditions at the airport were so bad. I wondered if this was a sign of things to come and struggled home at midnight to sleep, ready for the interview next day.

Chapter 13 — The Highlands

The morning after I had finished working in London, I travelled down to Inverness for the interview. Throughout the 50-minute journey, I practised how I would deliver the PowerPoint presentation, outlining my thoughts on managing the challenges and opportunities for the dietetic team. Armed with my trusty memory stick, I arrived for my interview at Raigmore Hospital just after lunchtime. I was quite a sight, smelling strongly of menthol cough sweets and sporting a nose that wouldn't have looked out of place on Santa's favourite reindeer! Somehow, I made it through my slides and answered a wide range of questions from the three panel members in turn. I was the only candidate but couldn't wait for it all to be over and I could only think of getting home and into bed. However, they asked me to wait in a side room while they considered my fate and, a short while later, I was ushered back in to be informed, with some relief, that the post was mine if I wanted it. The job would allow me to permanently re-locate and focus more on my family while they needed me most. I was very fortunate to be able to formally start my new contract the following Monday and, therefore, protected my continuous NHS service record and pension. It gave me a chance to settle into life back north of the border and recover from my cold. I took 2 weeks' unpaid leave to allow for all the necessary references and NHS checks and started work as the chief dietitian at the hospital in mid-November 2006. There was no induction arranged for me, so I got on as best I could, trying to meet up with the key people I thought I'd most likely be working with. Everyone I met was very welcoming but shocked to hear that I was travelling 40 miles each way to work. However, they quickly realised that it was so much better for me than my previous daily commute into and around London. The drive to Raigmore Hospital took less than an hour, which was more than half as long as my previous journey in and out of Kent. I was also travelling through fantastic scenery, passing lots of wildlife, with relatively little traffic to navigate or delay me. My daughters settled into their primary four class easily, so all I needed to do was to sell my house in England and navigate the Scottish property system to buy a new house for us... simple!

I settled into work quickly and was fortunate to have a very supportive manager in the larger-than-life form of Ron Ward, a jovial Yorkshire man, the directorate manager for hospital clinical services. He had a very broad remit, covering AHP services as well as laboratory and diagnostic teams. He was always very encouraging to me and hugely positive about my past work experiences. Shortly after starting work at the hospital, he helped me submit a proposal at a meeting of the hospital management team to expand and improve the general dietetic working environment. Our department had outgrown the cramped main office, and it no longer had the space we needed to function effectively. It had often been hard for clinicians to concentrate on work or have private telephone conversations with patients and colleagues in peace. Many of us had to share computers and phone lines and there was little room for storage of the ever-increasing number of patient records. Our renal, home enteral feeding and diabetes dietitians were scattered round the hospital site, and we lacked space for team meetings or to accommodate students on placement as the office quickly became overcrowded. The senior management team not only supported my request for new, larger office space, but they also funded re-decoration, new IT hardware for everyone, air conditioning and separate out-patient clinic facilities. It was a big boost for us all and, when the move came, we had great support from our estates and teams of porters who helped us relocate in just a few hours.

I reflected how much harder it would have been to implement such a smooth office move so quickly had I still worked in Kent, where it would have taken a huge amount of organisation and a long trail of paperwork to co-ordinate the whole process. Fellow AHP service managers were all very welcoming and we supported each other within our directorate team, delivering lots of positive service improvements. Working life in Highland NHS was certainly much more informal and laid back than I was used to in my previous role. I reflected to Ron that any service change appeared to happen at a glacial pace compared to what I had been used to in the hectic demands of the NHS in the southeast of England. I commented to several people that it felt as though I had gone into reverse gear. I found it very hard to adjust and slow down my work rate after years of a much faster pace and far tighter budgetary restrictions. It would be another twelve years before the health board invested in a dedicated project management team to take a more robust managed process. The board was no different to many others, and we always seemed to have to get a grip on the recurring financial challenges of the day.

The team of dietitians were all very close friends outside of work and social lives merged into that.. It was sometimes hard to focus on what we were doing as other colleagues would also appear to collect post or file record cards. I gradually realised that this was a common feature of NHS Highland no matter whichever part of the organisation you worked in. Lots of people in the hospital were either related to, friends with, neighbours of or part of the same social activities as other staff and close colleagues. Our part-time secretary was managed through a general admin team manager and was a well-liked, key part of the department. Like most departments I've worked in, staff often confided their woes to her, and she became something of an agony aunt to the younger dietitians, particularly when romance was involved. I was grateful for her willingness to adapt and take on all the changes to the department, including a move to digital dictation, which saved everyone lots of time. It also meant that she no longer had to try and decipher everyone's handwritten notes.

I gradually settled in and adjusted to my daily commute and my role in Inverness, trying to manage and support the staff and services of the department. As with many other young teams, several staff were already in serious romantic relationships, and one was busy planning her wedding, with two colleagues as bridesmaids. I was invited to join staff, past and present, to a pre-wedding celebration at a local city-centre restaurant, so I made the extra effort to be there by arranging a babysitter for my daughters and travelled back down to Inverness again one evening. It was a good way of getting to know people informally and to meet others no longer working at Raigmore. However, unbeknown to any of us, someone had arranged a surprise for the bride-to-be, and during our dinnertime conversation, events were overtaken by the arrival of a young man and his girlfriend. To the horror of many, he turned out to be a male stripper and she was his assistant... sitting in the background playing his musical accompaniment on her CD player! I don't know who was more shocked or embarrassed, but it never happened again when any of the others went on to get married.

Career opportunities in very rural organisations are generally few and far between once people settle down and build a family. Highland was no different and I came across many staff who had stayed in the same role/team/location for many years — entire careers, in lots of cases. I wasn't used to this in any of my previous workplaces and found it quite a strange situation. I was used to appointing people from all over the country, and found that they offered more experience, better practice and insights from other departments. Having moved around the English NHS so often over the years, I couldn't imagine that I would ever have had access to the same opportunities or be promoted through professional ranks nearly as quickly if I had remained close to home after qualifying from RGU. Many people find change difficult and unsettling, whereas I have always thrived on it. I like to network, innovate and think out of the box and have always believed that there are many chances to do things differently. Sometimes that can mean an unconventional approach but that's often necessary when transforming the way we deliver services, and ensures we deliver high-quality, safe care to people.

In April 2007, a great opportunity came up to work in Morayshire as the local dietetic manager, also the BDA Hon. Chair, Judith Catherwood, had left for a new post with NHS Education Scotland (NES). I was tipped off about the vacancy by a colleague in Aberdeen, noting that there was only a week until the closing date. I had only been at work in Inverness for a few months but my mother's health had continued to deteriorate and she was in and out of hospital a lot, so any opportunity to stay closer to home would have been helpful. I suspected that they might have an internal candidate in mind for the job but decided to try my best anyway and continued to work through the application process. On the day of the interview, I arrived in the waiting area just as the first, and only other internal candidate came out chatting and laughing with the hospital manager — the chair of the panel. I was ushered in afterwards and met the other two people ready to interview me, one from HR along with the dietetic head of service in Aberdeen. I was pleased with how I answered all the questions and was my usual "glass half full" upbeat self throughout. It was obvious, however, that the hospital manager had already made her mind up about who she wanted, and she stared at me expressionlessly as I smiled and enthusiastically answered all her questions. When it was the turn of the HR officer, she beamed at me and announced, "I really want you to be my life coach —

you're so positive!" Despite all that, it was no surprise to me when I took a phone call later that afternoon from the hospital manager. She explained that I hadn't been successful and that I just wasn't "the right fit!" It was the first time in seventeen years that I'd failed to get a job that I'd applied for, but with hindsight, I thought she was right; my "glass half full" outlook was never going to fit.

Talking with staff in one-to-ones back in Inverness, many commented that they were keen to develop themselves and their roles. I could see lots of potential to grow a great service and for them to have a higher profile in the national world of dietetics. Until then, they had generally not been encouraged to look outwards from the board area or network more widely. They seemed keen to try new ideas and be more innovative, either on their own or as a team. For all the years I had worked in England with the BDA, I also had a pretty good idea, through the extensive IR network of meetings, conferences and news, of what was happening in Scotland. However, there had never really been a high-profile name in Highland, apart from

Judith Catherwood, who lived there but worked in NHS Grampian. I had previously been very immersed in, and surrounded by, colleagues who supported BDA work over the years. So, I was very taken aback to notice that the professional association had little or no profile in our wider team at the time. Record-keeping and clinical standards that had been developed and adopted in other areas of the UK over many years still hadn't been implemented across the Highland team. However, we soon agreed that we would start to embed them into practice, at least within our hospital-based acute team. The community dietetic service was not part of my remit and comprised of a very limited, uncoordinated group of several part-time staff, scattered across the extensive board area. I was pleased to see a familiar face from Kent, who was now based on Skye, and proactively delivering single-handed service there. Others did well to deliver a range of clinical services across quite remote localities within the limitations of their part-time roles but there was little cover for any absences. The current situation is much improved, but recruitment has always been a challenge in community services, especially in the more remote areas. There was a concern that if posts were left vacant too long, it would prove the vacant post was no longer needed and money could potentially be removed from budgets. They were managed by local general managers and were able to access over-arching professional advice from the head of service. Our specialist colleagues, based at Raigmore, offered support and training for them and they would often contact us wanting our help and advice. I've continued to believe that we all have a role to play in supporting people to reflect and understand their contribution with the wider team. We started to have more clinical update days to learn more about each other's roles and specialist areas, which also helped inform and motivate staff, as well as students on placement.

Early in 2007, we decided to organise a Raigmore team-building day, which would help us get to know each other better, to reflect on each other's strengths and to make some plans for the year ahead. We were only able to organise this for hospital dietetic staff but

Ron supported me to bring an external facilitator, Jean Balfour, up from Kent. I had firsthand experience of her successful models of away-days for PEC, Board and organisational teams and this one was no exception. The event in Inverness was really good fun and staff appreciated the time out. There was also a sense that Ron and I were investing the time and effort in them, listening to their views on what needed to change for the better. Recruiting staff to such a remote and rural area was always challenging so it felt right that we created an encouraging environment for each other. That would make it easier to create a supportive friendly team with a good reputation and help to retain our staff.

Early in my career in Inverness, I found myself back in familiar territory when Ron asked me to take over as the organisational lead for the management of the home enteral feeding contract. I had stumbled across a potential missed saving of £35k — a significant proportion of the budget for NHS Highland. It wasn't nearly as large as the contracts that I'd previously led in England so I was happy to fit it into my workload. We moved on from a situation where there had been small lunchtime meetings with a company representative, in a local restaurant, to the more formal footing that I was used to with a broad mix of clinicians, procurement and finance colleagues. There was lots of tidying up to do to make sure that the board didn't lose out anymore and to check that we were getting the best value for money. Ron and our board nurse director both made it clear that they were delighted to know that it was now being well-managed. We were happy to see reps from all companies, who kept us up to date with new products and services. One of them was Jan, my best friend from RGU days, who had moved out of NHS dietetics some years previously. We both knew that our paths would cross at work from the moment I got the job and both declared our friendship early on to avoid any complaints about potential conflicts of interest. I was relieved to find that there was good nursing support for patients requiring home enteral feeding, as the board area we covered was so vast. An electronic patient registration and management system was gradually introduced, helping us to support patients and clinical staff respond to any type of feeding problems or changes. Several years later, a nursing app was introduced, allowing patients faster access to support, which prevented potential delays in treatment and unnecessary hospital admissions. One of the best aspects of contract tendering and scrutiny in Scotland is the centralised joined-up approach, which is co-ordinated and led by the national procurement team. They take all the stress out of the process for clinicians, and company representatives too, and arranged round-table discussions of Board representatives for the planning and monitoring of contracts. It was also a good way for me to link up with colleagues from other areas, and, with dietetics being the profession it is, we were often already acquainted from working together on some BDA committee or project over the years. The professional network is important to help us all understand and learn from each other's work, to avoid duplication and to build new and existing working relationships. It also helped me to build my own understanding of the key policies, people and plans that would be important to my career, as I was still getting to grips with the structures and policies in NHS Scotland.

In 2007, I took the opportunity of contacting the healthcare manager at HMP Inverness and, after explaining my interest and experiences in England, he invited me to visit him and showed me round the healthcare department and the general prison environment. It was tucked behind an unremarkable row of residential houses not far from the Inverness courthouse and was quite a bit smaller than the huge prisons I'd been used to working with in London and the southeast of England. Unusually, it housed a mix of young offenders and adult inmates — remand and sentenced men — as well as having a small separate area for women. On the day I visited, there were two staying there and both were fully occupied with cleaning duties. I was shown around the wings and the compact kitchen area where a mix of prisoners and officers were preparing lunch for the day. An old prisoner wandered past, apparently confused about where he was. He asked a prison officer, "Am I in the wrong shed?" He was directed to his cell in the neighbouring wing and toddled off unsteadily. Meanwhile, our attention was diverted to the sound of a young man banging on his cell door, complaining of having a sore head. The irony of the noise he was creating wasn't lost on the staff and he was told quite firmly that he wasn't at home now and to lie down quietly. In line with prison rules, he wouldn't be getting paracetamol until the medical centre was open after lunchtime. Healthcare in Scottish prisons was still the responsibility of the Scottish Prison Service at that time but that would gradually change to mirror the English model that I'd been used to, as the local NHS teams gradually took over responsibility a few years later, allowing easier access to more local community-based clinicians who started to visit more regularly.

I was keen to explore how I could use some of my other skills and knowledge locally and wondered whether local football clubs might want to invest in sports nutrition advice. I contacted the manager at Caledonian Thistle — the only premier division club in the area at the time — but sadly they weren't interested. I was undeterred though and contacted

1st division club Ross County, in the nearby town of Dingwall. I was really encouraged to be invited to visit and talk with the manager and find out more about the club, players and catering facilities. We explored the possibility of the club paying NHS Highland for me to deliver a training session to players and coaching staff, and shortly afterwards, I was asked along to spend the day talking with them about the potential impact of good sports nutrition and hydration. Some of the young players also brought their landladies along because many of them were staying a long way from their families, dependent on having meals provided for them. It was clearly important that their nutritional requirements were being catered for to give them the best chance of maximising their playing potential. I'd already established that many of their dietary habits were quite poor, compounded by trips to the local supermarket, where they stocked up on many unhealthy food choices. The training and discussions were a great success, resulting in both players and landladies now much more interested in making positive changes to their eating habits. The club took my suggestions on board too and started to make healthier food choices more available at lunchtimes and on match days. They also continued to use my PowerPoint presentation to reinforce the key messages to others who hadn't been to the training session. I was delighted to see that they were promoted to the premier division the following year, though I'm not taking any personal credit for that. It was almost certainly down to the quality and commit- ment of players and staff. I can only hope that their understanding of the transformational role that good hydration and nutrition can have on performance might have been a positive contributory factor.

Like many other departments, our team at Raigmore Hospital supported student dietitians on placement from three Scottish universities. In the spring of 2007, I discovered that we were scheduled to be routinely inspected on behalf of the Health Professions Council (HPC). Unusually, my job description didn't require me to have the board lead for organising local place- ments. However, I was managing the dietitian who did most of the hands-on co-ordination of them. I was delighted to see that our "inspector" was Fiona, a colleague from Edinburgh, who I'd known for many years through various BDA connections. She greeted me with a warm hug and we had a quick catch up about student training before she was whisked away. Her day was planned out for her, meeting with various other clinicians and managers to hear their perspectives about the dietetic team and training commitments in the hospital. We caught up at the end of the day and I was delighted that we received a very positive report. Student training in the Highlands continued to gradually evolve over the years and now, all dietitians working in every care setting are involved, rather than just a few as in the early days. The HCPC no longer routinely carry out on-site inspections for new or existing placements as all staff are expected to participate in training the new generation of clinicians regardless of the hours and in whichever speciality they work. As I have reflected from my own personal experience, students really benefit from time in the community, hospital and various clinical environments. To pass their placements, they must demonstrate evidence of clinical knowledge, professionalism and communication skills. It's no longer just the domain of hospital staff, and novel placements now include the armed services, sports teams and even the BDA office.

As any NHS manager knows, working as part of a young female-dominated profession can have its challenges. One is the implementation of family-friendly policies and the unknown quantity of requests for maternity leave, carers' leave and other similar time away from work. As a manager, it can be quite a juggling act to make sure that the needs of the service are covered with adequate staffing ratios and clinical experience. I had started with just 13 qualified staff in 2006 and, at one point, we had four women off on maternity leave. Coupled with a vacancy and people needing to take their annual leave and support study leave, it was quite a challenge to recruit junior staff to backfill their posts, but somehow, we did. I think we did well to be able to offer them a good mix of experience and opportunities to develop their careers. Our department grew larger as we received more funding, allowing us to employ more dietetic assistants as well as specialist staff. In a few years, we soon had twenty-two in the team, which created a challenge in finding desk space for everyone. We were fortunate to have access to the Centre for Health Sciences building across the site — a fairly modern, spacious building with good opportunities for the use of digital technology.

I think it is vital for managers to support staff to fulfil their potential and to plan ahead for career succession in the future. I took the opportunity to develop a structure of several specialist clinical teams — paediatric, diabetic, renal and acute — delegating management responsibility to the team leads and setting up senior team meetings, allowing them to further develop organisational skills and those related managing staff and budgets. For many managers, the focus was much more about having lots of senior staff, but like me, our new associate director of AHP services (Judith Catherwood) was keen for all AHP teams to have a 65:35 ratio of qualified to unqualified staff and we hit it exactly. I'm a firm believer that we should only be using valuable staff time and expertise for the clinical experience that they're trained to deliver. Any other administrative work and associated support should be delivered by secretarial or healthcare assistant roles. This not only allows team budgets to be used more effectively but it also improves job satisfaction and staff retention.

Despite the challenges of being a manager, I continued to focus on doing my best and Judith encouraged me to stretch my skill set even further. A new NHS Scotland uniform had been developed and there was a clear expectation that all boards would roll it out within a tight timescale. I was asked to co-ordinate the approach for the implementation of this across the entire Raigmore Hospital site, making sure that everyone knew which colours and styles were to be used for each professional speciality. It went well and she was delighted with the outcome, as all staff groups successfully adopted the new uniforms, in turn, and on time. She was also keen for us to develop a plan to demonstrate the need to invest in a prescribing dietetic role and asked me to prepare a proposal, referencing all the evidenced work from my extensive experience in England. It was approved by the Board and we were able to recruit to a short-term post, funded from a community enteral feeding rebate scheme that was already in place. We all have a broad range of skills and expertise that should be nurtured and developed, regardless of our job titles. By allowing staff to develop their careers and try new opportunities, the wider organisation also benefits. Good leaders enjoy seeing staff stretch their wings and fly, while others feel threatened and prefer to retain an iron grip control, which is stifling and leads to staff who are unable to fulfil their potential. I've seen a range of all over the years and Highland was certainly no different.

Judith went on to accept an opportunity to pick up a new personal career challenge in Australia and she made a life-changing decision to move across the world to become an executive AHP director in Brisbane. Thankfully, for me, Katherine Sutton, a radiographer by background, was appointed into the role soon after. I was relieved that her approach was very encouraging to all staff in her wider team, walking the walk of good leadership. The only thing that is constant in any large public organisation like the

NHS is change. My experience of NHS Highland is no different and, as a result, I have lived through several re-organisations and numerous comings and goings in management and professional advisors above me. At various times and overlapping at different times, during my time there, I had 8 different line managers, 3 AHP leads, 4 AHP directors and 1 professional lead. To add to the confusion, not everyone agreed with what each other wanted from me at the same time, making it quite confusing and conflicting at times. However, my role continued to develop, and I went on to become the dietetic services manager for both the hospital and surrounding community areas. At Raigmore, it was good to see that we now had a much better-staffed department, offering a range of job opportunities for staff grades and roles spanning pay bands 2-7. There were now four team lead roles, each with their own mix of staff skills and grades to manage and develop. However, in 2012, a paper was presented to the senior management team, proposing that NHS Highland no longer needed to employ dietetic staff above a band 7 level. This resulted in my post — the only band 8 dietetic role in the board — being dis-established the following year. I can only imagine that other AHP teams were worried that it might set a trend in their areas. Over time, of course, it became clear that this had been a very short-sighted view, adversely impacting on dietetic career progression opportunities, the ability to offer strong service leadership, and the experience to deliver transformational change across Highland. The BDA has always advocated having a career structure that supports staff development, including management grades, to provide strong, senior leadership. As NHS Highland and Highland Council moved forward to create a ground-breaking lead agency model, the paediatric dietitians soon moved out of the health board into local authority management structures, now focused on supporting children and families. The remaining band-7 team leads left their posts and the structure failed due to the lack of service investment and management expertise, which was sad to witness. However, I received support and encouragement from board and senior management members,

and I was able to take advantage of the local redeployment policy. Not for the first time in my career, a
new and exciting opportunity allowed me to move
on to pastures new.

Chapter 14 — New beginnings

By the spring of 2014, NHS Highland had taken on the lead agency role for all adult health and social care services. Reports shared with board directors demonstrated that nutritional care was an area that was being regularly raised as a significant and consistent concern in care inspectorate reports of care homes in the Highlands. I was delighted when Nigel, my operational manager, and Katherine Sutton — by now the associate director of AHPs — approached me with the offer of a brand-new role allowing me to transition across to Board HQ, into the adult social care team, with the same terms and conditions of service. The job description for nutrition and dietetic advisor for care homes was perfect for my skill set and appeared to be just the sort of strategic post I had always relished. Working as part of the senior social work team was fascinating and opened my eyes to another world of caring for vulnerable people. NHS Highland now owned 16 adult care homes but had responsibility for dozens more, many privately owned by individuals or larger companies. Historically, they had had little contact with dietetic staff, other than to see individual residents for clinical advice. There had been no co-ordination of nutritional care training and staff relied on a range of websites or other sources to get advice.

It was a completely unique role for the UK dietetic profession with lots of potential to explore, innovate and network much more widely than I had been able to do at Raigmore Hospital. They wanted me to take a fresh look at food, fluid and nutrition care within adult social care services and develop the role, using my extensive range of contacts and insights. I was encouraged to take an enquiring approach, considering how I could positively influence all aspects of residents' lives and limitations of staff knowledge. I couldn't have been happier as it played to all my strengths, giving me the opportunity to deliver service transformation, freedom to shape and develop existing and new professional networks, and to have the autonomy to use my initiative. I had a very positive working partnership with both Nigel and Katherine, who both expected and trusted me to work with light-touch supervision, which is what I had always been used to prior to working in the Highlands. I was also delighted to be able to take responsibility for the board-wide enteral feeding contract with me from my previous post. At the time, I was the only member of dietetic service who had the experience to manage it through an imminent re-tendering exercise. Linked to that was the lead professional role for nutritional product prescribing, which remained a significant gap in the Highland dietetic service. Three months into the post, I met with Nigel and Katherine again so that I could report on my progress. They couldn't believe all the network connections that I'd made or how much I had managed to achieve in such a short space of time. In Nigel's words, "I don't know why we didn't develop this post before; there's so much to do!" Katherine then invited me to join the Highland-wide AHP leadership team, which she chaired, to help develop strategic direction for all the relevant professions across the board area.

I was really pleased and reassured to have been met with strong support from all the care home managers who I'd met during my induction period. They were really appreciative of now having dietetic input and welcomed my offers of training and advice to help them with inspection reports. One afternoon in the summer of 2014, I had the opportunity to visit an independent care home in Ross-shire. Having been taken over by Parklands Group, it was in the process of upgrading its facilities by moving to a brand-new building next door. The external building looked very tired and run down but as I walked through the main entrance, I realised how appearances can be deceptive because it seemed to be a great place to live and work. As I waited to meet Denise, the manager, I was able to observe the lovely caring atmosphere in the dining area as staff helped with the meal service. It was warm and friendly with lots of positive interaction between everyone there. When I sat down with Denise and her senior team, I realised why everything was so nice.

They clearly had a genuine fondness for their service users and were excited about moving into the new building next door, which would improve the general environment and facilities for staff and service users living and working there. We would go on to have a long, respectful working relationship, which delivered many service and care improvements for people in the home. Our work also led to positive developments for other parts of the country as we went on to have great success.

Using the same model as my previous work in burns and spinal injuries specialities, I thought it would be helpful to be able to link in with other colleagues across Scotland who were also providing some dietetic services to care home settings. With the help of a colleague in the Care Inspectorate, we gathered a group of about a dozen community dietitians from a range of Scottish health boards, at Perth Royal Infirmary. This began a long-lasting, supportive professional collaboration. Twice yearly meetings and regular contact allowed us to jointly develop and share resources, experiences and plans to improve food, fluid and nutrition in social care settings.

I was asked to take on the role of chair for the first year and we agreed to rotate the role each subsequent year to give everyone the chance to share the responsibility and develop their own planning and organisational skills. The group continued to meet twice a year and we became a great support to each other, discussing examples of our practice and planning a consistent, once for Scotland approach. Alison Molyneux (Glasgow), Hazel Rogers (Tayside), Pamela Weir (Lanarkshire), Gail Devine (Forth Valley) and Caroline Berry (Fife) were there from the start, although membership has since changed and the group continues to invite others to join in. I encouraged them to focus particularly on managing the increasing risk of swallowing problems faced by many of our residents and we all co-ordinated a consistent, joined-up programme for nutrition and hydration week in spring 2018. By the summer of 2019, we had developed an agreed protocol for auditing staff hydration in our care homes. Eight out of 14 boards took part and the results were shared more widely to encourage staff to improve their own hydration.

In the summer of 2014, I had organised the first of many texture modification training days for social care staff working across the Highlands. In all my discussions with care home managers, this was the area of practice and care which was causing them most concern in trying to safely support people who had a swallowing difficulty (dysphagia). I developed a very interactive programme with contributions from a variety of speakers, including speech therapy, occupational therapy and a well-known demonstration chef with a reputation for fun, engaging presentations. In future years, we would also go on to include oral health educators and other inspirational care chefs. In the seven years that I ran them, the evaluations from staff and speakers were — and continued to be — hugely positive. Some participants were quite overcome by how much better texture modified meals could be and several left the first session close to tears, realising that their residents must be enduring very poor experiences at mealtimes. They were determined to put their learning into practice and improve the lives of the people in their care. We continued to run three or four sessions a year and they were always well-attended and evaluated by people working in a wide range of community and residential settings. From my early experience, social care staff and managers were like enthusiastic sponges; desperate for new learning and development opportunities to be delivered in a very practical format. There had previously been little investment in their nutritional training needs from community dietetics so the new model of adult health and care in Highland really helped to address their learning gaps. The nature of the work meant that many homes had a high staff turnover and all new starters needed to be kept up to date with evidenced-based information. Sitting in front of PowerPoint presentations for hours didn't suit their busy lives and learning styles so we used fun, new educational tools like the Dysphagia game (@Focus games) which created informal, relevant learning with added competition and lots of laughter between care staff who came from all over the Highlands. This work transformed the way that care staff and cooks supported residents living with dysphagia to eat safely and well. As people continue to live longer, with neurological conditions such as dementia, MND, Parkinson's disease and the effects of strokes, the need for close focus and attention in delivering safe, varied mealtimes and snacks has become even more important.

During the summer of 2014, I was introduced to my new manager when NHS Highland appointed Joanna MacDonald as the Director of adult social care. Her auburn hair and boundless energy made her stand out from the crowd; like a breath of fresh air with a hint of Tigger about her! She always greeted people with a bright beaming smile, interested to listen to everyone's views and encourage their work. Her heels were vertiginous, but it didn't stop her always being on the go, spinning lots of plates, full of dogged determination to raise standards for service users across all social care settings. She made it clear, to those of us in her senior team, that she trusted us completely as professionals to do our jobs well and gave us all the autonomy and flexibility to work with minimal supervision. She included me in her senior team meetings and development sessions but always knew what we were working on and when to offer support if needed. There are less than a dozen people in my career — mostly women — who have made a strong impression as inspirational leaders and she quickly became one of them. Working alongside Katherine Sutton in 2014/15, the two of them really helped raise my confidence again and continued to encourage me to network widely with national partners. This helped to raise the profile of my unique role and shine a light on the important work being developed and delivered in our social care settings.

An unexpected opportunity presented itself when I heard that NES were looking for dietitians to collaborate with them and develop and evaluate social care placements for students assigned to health boards. I immediately responded, knowing exactly which care home manager I would approach for help – Denise. She jumped at the chance as did Dr Myra MacKenzie, a senior lecturer from RGU, with whom I went on to build a great partnership over the years. My mind was full of possibilities of all the experiences we could offer students. There were also several projects that would help raise the profile of nutritional care and help them gather evidence for their university portfolios.

The Raigmore dietetic team was seriously under-staffed and struggling to deliver core clinical services at the time, so offering to support student placements took a lot of pressure off them and went down very positively. Emma, the local dietetics student training lead, and Kerrie, Highland's AHP practice education lead, were also keen to explore them with us. It wasn't long before we had an opportunity to meet and talk through all the ideas and practicalities of implementing them. We were joined on-line by Edith McIntosh from the Care Inspectorate and Karen Allen from NES. Our first social care placement was piloted in October 2014 and was a huge success for all concerned. It had required good, detailed forward planning, helped by having an enthusiastic and very capable mature final-year student from RGU. The skills and willingness of The Parkland's team to embark on a ground-breaking venture allowed us to deliver another first in the world of UK dietetics. Katherine, our student, carried out a variety of projects but one stood out above all and is still talked about today: "Rabbit stew, anyone?" One afternoon, she sat down with the activities co-ordinator and a group of residents who were living with varying stages of dementia. She planned to talk with them about their memories of life during the Second World War and particularly their memories of food rationing and mealtimes. None of us knew whether the residents would engage or what they might say but one lady, whose dementia was quite advanced, suddenly started to describe how she used to walk to the village butcher with her mum to buy a fresh rabbit, which was hanging over the shop front. Her mum would take it home and skin it, clean the skin and then, the following week, sell it for a penny to a man who came round the houses. She then used it to pay for her food shopping the following week. To say that the hairs on the back of my neck stood up was an understatement but the lady's daughters were equally stunned, having never heard the story of their mum's wartime childhood before. As a direct result of this conversation, the recollections of the eight residents' wartime meals were transformed into a special menu for a World War Two celebration that Denise's team planned for the entire home and visiting relatives. It consisted of Scotch broth, rabbit stew and clootie dumpling and everyone loved it.

Staff dressed up as land girls, and wartime music played in the background, which many sang along to. It was great for the residents and the families who joined in but I was especially pleased for Katherine who had been able to see her initial conversation translate into a very successful outcome for all. Never let it be said that people with dementia can't be involved in menu-planning. Using reminiscence conversations, it's perfectly possible to understand what people would enjoy eating or drinking routinely, or for special occasions, before building these into mealtime options. Our work was shortlisted for an AHP Advancing Healthcare award in early 2015 and we were delighted to have reached the final three from our category. Denise and I attended the ceremony in London one afternoon in April 2015. It was full of glitz and glamour and all the

chief health professions officers from the home countries were there. I was pleased to see representatives
from every professional association, including the
Honorary Chairman of the BDA. We were more than
happy to be runners-up to the winner of our category
who went on to be the overall winner of winners on
the day. All the Scottish finalists celebrated together
and were invited for a group photo with Scotland's
(then) chief health professions officer, Jacqui Lundy,
and her deputy, Tracy MacInnes.

I was incredibly proud and delighted when our new
model of social care placements was also awarded the
prestigious Dame Barbara Clayton Award at the 2015
BDA conference. Emma and I flew down to the awards
ceremony just a few hours after I had completed
another successful day of care home training. It was
refreshing and enjoyable to meet up with many
familiar colleagues, including Morag Mackellar, a
past Hon. Chairman — who I had sat alongside at
many previous BDA council meetings — in her role
as awards coordinator. She had overseen the judging
of our submission and presented trophies to us all

after a great conference dinner, catching up with old acquaintances and making new connections. Morag is another inspirational colleague who has also gone on to receive an OBE and she continues to be an inspirational AHP leader in NHS Forth Valley, working into her 8th decade!

Later in the summer, we went on to enter this successful "rabbit stew" experience for a Scottish dementia award, focusing on our unique partnership work. We were over the moon to be shortlisted as finalists in our category once again. Denise, Myra, Katherine and I made the journey to the awards ceremony along with Muriel, the cook, and Ron Taylor, the owner of the Parklands Care Group. We were more than happy to receive a runners-up certificate, which we all proudly promoted widely throughout our various organisations. We continued to adapt and develop the model for social care placements for students at all stages of training, in both care home and social care teams. Our experiences and examples of developing them subsequently encouraged other teams across the UK to expand the range of locations of their placements into social care. The students always really enjoyed spending time during these weeks and they often commented on the very different social model of care, which is far more person-centred than the structured clinical model in the busy ward environment of most healthcare settings. They had time to sit down to chat, getting to know residents, who always enjoyed having new people showing an interest in them and the chance for fresh conversation. I also started writing "Nutrition News" early in 2015, aimed at supporting and sharing learning among social care staff and services across The Highlands. It continued to be a very popular, well-evaluated quarterly publication until I retired at the end of 2021. We all have very different learning styles and for practical, personal reasons, covering 70 care homes, the option of face-to-face training just isn't a viable or cost-effective option. The newsletter had a large circulation across the Highlands and was also shared across many groups and national agencies in Scotland. Links were sent out via social media too, which had a far greater reach than I could ever have achieved on my own. I felt very fortunate to be able to spend time talking with many of our residents and was always interested to hear about their fascinating lives and experiences growing up in the Highlands. Profiling them (with their permission) and their daily routines in Nutrition News created lots of interest for people who have never set foot in a care home before, changing perceptions about older people and their lives. I have interviewed many interesting people with so many fascinating backgrounds. One unassuming lady had her MBE proudly on display in her room, another man described his many years as an archaeologist, there were nurses who had worked in the Highlands, while others who shared wartime stories of rural life. They are always delighted to see themselves in print and it creates a great talking point for their families and fellow residents in their homes. Colleagues from many other professions — including AHPs, specialist nurses and consultants — were willing to contribute articles about their specialist areas of work, and social care staff benefitted from sharing examples of activities and what they were doing locally, which was a great way of both motivating others and learning together.

I was delighted when Myra later introduced me to her colleagues, and I was invited to go back to RGU to talk about my role and encourage students to consider placements in social care. It brought back memories of the hospital dietitian who had come to speak to us in the mid-80s. Thirty years later, however, I had no need for a white coat or a nasogastric tube around my neck.

Back in the Highlands, I was now involved in a new project, working with Focus games to develop a new Hydration board game. The University of East Anglia, and Caroline Lecko from patient safety England (previously with me at NPSA), were also involved and I was able to try out the prototypes with care home staff and residents from three different settings. To see the final versions was a real highlight and a great addition to a suite of learning and development tools that social care and other staff could make effective use of, even involving residents and their families for some fun. I continued to work with the team at Focus to develop and try out new games to use as educational tools. The Dysphagia game was one of the most useful, given the large number of care home residents who required adapted food and fluids to keep them safe and well-nourished. During Covid, the games were made digitally available, which allowed for ongoing training, especially helpful for new care staff and cooks.

In my day job, I was frequently asked by social work colleagues to offer support and advice during large scale investigations into care homes that were struggling to deliver the standard of care that their residents should have expected. There was often a lack of effective leadership, difficulty recruiting and retaining staff — including cooks — putting lots of very frail vulnerable people at risk when they should have expected to feel safe, well cared for and valued in their final years. Many homes simply didn't improve care to the required level. They were subsequently shamed publicly and forced to close sending a clear message to relatives and service users that NHS Highland expected far higher standards for all service users. The learning from these situations is often helpful in supporting others to move forward. Managers were very clear that they needed to ensure mealtimes were enjoyable, person-centred, varied and safe. There was a heightened understanding about the important key role of cooks and carers in offering appropriate texture modified diets. I believe that this created an increasing appreciation for the essential role played by care caterers and encouraged care staff to include them in staff meetings and care planning discussions. We all know how a poor mealtime experience can spoil our holidays or stay in hospital so we need to truly understand the potentially harmful impact on our residents, who totally depend on staff to deliver a safe, enjoyable choice of food and drinks, which they can look forward to each day. I was invited to speak at national meetings of the Scottish HCA to share and discuss ideas so that we could develop a more consistent approach to a safe, nutritious meal service. I also worked closely with care inspectorate colleagues, at local and national level, to develop consistent messaging and reliance on an evidence base for good nutritional care. I was pleased to be invited to deliver a workshop alongside Joyce Murray, the head of health improvement, at their national conference in Dunblane in early 2016.

I arrived one Sunday evening, having driven down the A9 through terrible blizzard conditions, and went straight to bed. The next day was a buzz of activity, and I met the friendly, familiar faces of Edith MacIntosh, Heather Edwards and Jackie Dennis who were always really encouraging of my work in social care settings.

There was a great turnout with video conference links to delegates who had been unable to attend, including some from the far reaches of NHS Highland, which was nice to see. The focus of the event was promoting continence, an area where nutritional care has a big part to play. One speaker — a care home manager — spoke of the great success her staff had seen in gradually weaning residents off laxatives, which had often been started before admission to the home. Proactively assisting improved hydration had transformed the lives of many residents who had become socially isolated, depressed and struggled to control their bowel movements. Once gradually weaned off laxatives, they became happier, healthier, more engaged in activities, mixing with others and eating better. I continue to share this message at all opportunities during teaching sessions in my day job, writing blogs and encouraging a transformational approach to promoting continence. Over the coming year, I worked with the health improvement team, in consultation with a range of clinicians, agencies and social care colleagues, to develop a "once for Scotland" food and fluid resource for elderly care settings. It was launched in late 2017 and now sits within the care inspectorate improvement hub, along with YouTube clips of me and others including care chefs, an advisor for Scottish Care and a few care home managers. To date, it is one of my proudest achievements. I remain passionate about ensuring our old and vulnerable service users are given every opportunity to eat well and stay well, enjoying mealtimes with a wide selection of food and drinks that they would choose themselves. Working with Alzheimer Scotland's lead AHP and the wider team also helped highlight the importance of engaging positively with many service users who lacked mental capacity. I continued to enjoy a positive working relationship with Professor Elaine Hunter until retirement.

Never being one to sit still, I enjoyed having several projects on the go at the same time. During the autumn of 2016, a new challenge presented itself when we were struggling to really get to grips with escalating costs of prescribing oral nutritional supplements. It was hard to understand the true extent of the spending, as the data at the time was so variable and not easy to compare. I was invited to join a Scottish government working group, representing NHS Highland, alongside colleagues from dietetics and pharmacy from other health boards. It's a small world really and many were already known to each other through our work on the enteral feeding contract for Scotland. The national work was driven forward by the chair, Janie Gordon, and we developed it further locally with the support and expertise of well-motivated people from a variety of clinical teams. The Highland prescribing group took some very "brave" decisions, which were quite radical and challenging for those who were more risk-averse than us. We started by asking for all prescribing of nutritional supplements to stop in care homes. So many of the supplements were either not appropriate or had ended up in the bin anyway, as residents often didn't want to take them. Some required thickened products or had been given several weeks' supply of a flavour that they didn't like. Using a "food first" approach, cooks and care staff were encouraged to make good use of higher-calorie and protein-richer meals and snacks. They were able to work more closely with individuals, and, as you would at home, try to tempt them with smaller portions of their favourites. We all have foods that we turn to when we feel off colour and they're often much higher in calories than the food we usually eat. Have a think about yours.

Community clinicians were made aware of what we hoped to achieve and links to written information were shared widely to support anyone with a poor appetite. I was delighted with how we developed an agreed approach for prescribing for children, with good joint working between paediatric dietitians and pharmacists. In adult services, we also created a more standardised approach to management of gluten-free diets, infant milks/formulae and nutritional support. Many supermarkets now offer a far greater range and quality of gluten-free and other "free from" foods, certainly compared to when I first started out in my career. Prescribable products are often restricted to a limited list of what the health board will authorise for individuals and not everyone enjoys the taste or texture available. We encouraged clinicians to focus on conventional food and drinks that allowed a much wider variety of meals and snacks. The "food first" approach was well- received by health and social care staff and service users, sustainable going forward, and had saved the Board several hundred thousand pounds annually. We were now receiving regular standardised reports of prescribing, which we could examine down to individual patient level. It was good to be able to examine why people were getting certain products, and we were able to successfully challenge the need for them. Good governance is important from both a patient safety and financial aspect, but just as important, from a learning perspective. The health board started to develop a greater focus on transformational performance management. I was delighted to be included in the prescribing efficiencies work stream, incorporating a range of our nutrition-prescribing initiatives.

Early on in my career, someone once said to me that when you do something first, make sure you share it widely as no one remembers the people who come second or third. I was so proud of what we had all achieved together that I submitted poster abstracts for a variety of high-profile events. I was invited to present it at a European dietetic event — a first for me. EFAD (the European Federation of Dietetic Associations) was also celebrating their 40th anniversary at the conference in Rotterdam, which made it extra special. I was delighted to meet other colleagues from the BDA along with several colleagues from the past: Carole Middleton, from my time in Leeds, Alison McBride from RGU days and Pauline Douglas, famous for her work in promoting hydration. The world of dietetics is small indeed and I really enjoyed networking, sharing and making new links with others.

I submitted another application for an Advancing Healthcare award in early 2019 and was delighted to be invited to present our work to the judging panel. I was joined by Ian Rudd, director of pharmacy in Highland, who helped support me in answering the panel questions about the presentation. Thankfully, I had somehow managed to deliver it within the allotted 15-minute target and we got through the questions. We would have to wait for two months before finding out how we'd done, as the results were to be announced at the actual awards ceremony in central London later in the spring.

In April 2019, we arrived at the event, hosted in a large hotel near Victoria Station, and I saw that it was going to be as glitzy and glamorous as the last event I'd been at with Denise back in 2015. There was lots of social media activity and supportive messages from colleagues working across Scotland. We waited and hoped as we watched several other awards being handed over — then it was our turn…. There was huge applause and cheering at our table when it was announced that we had won our category! It had eluded me back in 2015 but that was a distant memory as I stepped forward with Ian to accept the trophy on behalf of the Highland nutrition prescribing team. It was presented by Tracy MacInnes on behalf of the Scottish Government. She had been with me at the 2015 ceremony when were runners-up, so it was even better because this time we were able to take home the trophy. Afterwards, Ian and I celebrated with Tracy, and social media went into meltdown with messages of congratulations from so many colleagues. The awards celebrate innovative, transformational work by AHPs and healthcare scientists. Delivering transformational change in a vast remote and rural geographical area has often had its detractors and challenges but there are also opportunities that more urban areas don't have. The trick is to find what works for the people you're trying to engage with and to deliver it using a variety of tools. In 2020, I was pleased to have abstracts selected by both the NES and the ICDA 2020 committee (International Confederation of Dietetic Associations), one in Edinburgh and the other in South Africa! My submissions had described the challenges to delivering effective educational opportunities in my social care work across the remote and rural Highlands. The Covid-19 pandemic meant both conferences were cancelled so the trips were postponed. However, it was good enough to know that others had independently considered our work to be worthy of national and international platforms.

From my time working in the prison health team, and the public sector leadership scheme, I have often taken the opportunity to write about aspects of my work and have encouraged others to share theirs. I continued writing for many national publications and, from 2018, was even commissioned to write a regular article about dietetics in social care settings for Network Health Digest (NHD). I also wrote for Highland publications, Dietetics Today, Care News and several blogs. I have found it very empowering, but also relaxing, to reflect on and share my insights of the profession from a variety of perspectives. I found it to be a great release to be given a voice — albeit on paper — and it was satisfying to receive very positive feedback, knowing that other people seemed to appreciate and enjoy the articles and the information I was sharing. They say that we all have a book in us and maybe all those articles were the platform I needed to move on with my ambition to become a writer in years to come.

Chapter 15 — The digital coming of age

The use of so many digital technologies and platforms has completely transformed the way we live, work and communicate now. It's a far cry from my RGU days when Dr Wise was showing us what a computer was and how it might help us in our future work. Today, we can barely function without all our gadgets, apps, technology and digital networks, both in our personal and work lives. The way that we all work and interact as clinicians has adapted and greatly benefitted our service users too. We have also become more confident in adopting and embracing new opportunities to develop our IT skills using a variety of new tools and software. Long gone are the days of acetate slides and coloured pens — thank goodness! Presentations are now routinely delivered using web-based platforms and links are made available to watch at our convenience.

I bought my first mobile phone in 1995 but didn't really know how to use it other than for phone calls. I didn't get a work one until 2001 and even then it was an old analogue (brick!) I had never really embraced all the possibilities technology had to offer, having lived through the age of screeching telephone IT connections, which were slow, cumbersome and hardly portable. Fast forward to 2015 and NES were keen to support NMAHPs (nurses, midwives and AHPs) to become confident digital leaders. They wanted us to motivate and encourage the local development of digitally enabled staff who could make better use of new and existing technologies. I didn't even have a smartphone at the time but I was getting used to using all the technology available to me and I was keen to challenge myself so I could develop my skills further. As a very rural health board, NHS Highland had very good access to video conferencing and staff were encouraged to use any available technology in practice. I was one of three people nominated to participate on behalf of NHS Highland for the 3rd cohort of the Scottish dNMAHP's programme. So, in another unforeseen turn of events, it became another transformational career opportunity that would lead to even greater things in my future career. On day one, we were introduced to the NHSS digital approach by Dr Lesley Holdsworth OBE, Scottish Government digital clinical lead, and Ann Rae from NES. They encouraged us to try out new technologies and to enthusiastically share our learning with colleagues back in our boards. One of the first tasks we had to complete was to set up a Twitter account and, not being particularly au fait with different social media platforms, I wasn't entirely sure how useful or relevant it would be for me — how times have changed! The first hurdle I had to get over was setting the account up on my laptop and I knew just the people to help me; my then 16-year-old twin daughters. They were horrified at the thought of me having my own Twitter account and couldn't believe that I would need to have my own one for work! One of them finally agreed to help me set it up on the strict understanding that I didn't follow her! Needless to say, we also agreed that she and her teenage friends wouldn't do the same to my professional account. After several months of linking in with other dNMAHP colleagues, we had built our confidence in using a variety of technologies and I felt happy enough to start sending my own tweets — although initially, I was supervised by another daughter! By 2016, I had secured my first smartphone at work and now had Twitter on the go. It completely transformed my life — once the teenagers showed me how to use it, of course! I discovered that it was now easier to find out about news and developments as they happened and didn't have to wait for things to cascade down tradi-tional organisational routes, which could take weeks, if they ever reached me at all.

I was now able to network far and wide, across borders, seas, organisations and professions at all levels. It was a perfect platform for my working style and it gave me a professional voice with opportuni-ties to share and promote aspects of working in social care and nutritional care that would otherwise have been impossible. My account went from strength to strength, and I was often surprised to see very senior, national figures following me and to have colleagues from the past get in touch, or to follow, re-tweet and like posts. I took the opportunity to share photos of my mobile Highland office (car) when I was travelling around the amazing scenery, visiting care homes in some very picturesque locations. However, I often struggled to get a phone signal or internet connection and would have to quickly pull over into a lay-by when the phone "pinged," indicating emails coming through a nearby mast. So many times, it happened when I was working in the most unlikely, remote places, giving me the chance to quickly check if I needed to change my plans or respond to something urgently.

There was never really an effective, formal way of developing dNMAHP within NHS Highland until the Covid crisis of 2020 forced everyone into social distancing and remote working, which required many more people to rapidly adopt the use of new technology. It helped, of course, that IT equipment suddenly became readily available from Covid-specific budgets. I continued to keep in touch with national developments after successfully finishing the cohort 3 programmes and actively encouraged others to maximise the benefits of setting up their own accounts. Over the coming years, many did and wished they'd engaged in social media platforms before. I wrote several articles about my ongoing digital journey and recounted many in a few national blogs. By the winter of 2019, I found myself being interviewed by Dr Lesley Holdsworth and two others, in a zoom meeting, for a place on the Scottish government's dNMAHP clinical leadership group, which was chaired by Debbie Proven, a well-known dietitian and respected Scottish government advisor. I was personally delighted to be appointed to the new position, but nothing compared to the praise I got from my daughters who had watched my digital journey with some bemusement. They even told their friends with a mixture of both pride and disbelief! I was now used to using Zoom, ECHO, VC meetings, various webinars, Go-To meetings and WhatsApp! I experienced another first in my career by delivering a webinar for Scotland's national dementia network team to around 150 people at the end of

2019. I shared the highs and lows of my experiences through the national AHPScot blog site, hoping to help others realise that they weren't alone and that it's okay if you don't always get things right first time. Sitting in my dining room one Friday, I watched nervously as the sky turned very black, wondering if my temperamental internet connection would hold and let me deliver a national webinar. Thankfully, it went without a hitch and helped me put to bed an awful previous experience when my screen went completely black and I had to try and deliver a presentation without being able to see the slides!

My digital journey continued into 2020 as "TEAMs" was rolled out during lockdown, giving me yet another platform to get to grips with. I noticed how much more tolerant people had become when colleagues struggled with technology. They were much more willing to share tips on how to use TEAMs backgrounds, deliver presentations and chair meetings — all very positive for productive meetings. My role with the Scottish government dNMAHP clinical leadership team continued to develop and, during the Covid pandemic, more isolated working arrangements were required. It meant a faster, wider rollout of many digital plat-forms and equipment, which would go on to become the "normal" way of doing business and supporting patients. Numerous webinars were generated to assist colleagues to make best use of them and try to continue to stay connected with work and keep up to date. The NHS will never be the same again and social care staff have had far greater investment in digital hardware and training than ever before. It was also a lifeline in allowing residents to keep in touch with family or friends when they were locked down, and for staff to connect remotely, avoiding so much travel or unnecessary face-to-face visits or training.

Chapter 16 — COVID

Sometime around the middle of March 2020, life for all of us changed beyond recognition. Preparing my training materials to head over to a care home on Skye the following day, I was approached by my manager. I was told that all staff would immediately be advised to work from home unless they were essential to clinical care. Access to care homes was to be heavily restricted to protect vulnerable residents, so all my plans were suddenly cancelled and my diary cleared. I packed up my trusty laptop and reference resources and drove home to begin a very different routine; waiting for further instructions about possible redeployment to support the Covid effort. I continued with my usual routine, starting work at 7.30 am, preferring to make the most of the quiet mornings so that I could finish earlier in the afternoon. I set about communicating offers of help, resources and advice to all my social care partners and national agencies and used the time to have a good old sort out of documents and emails that I'd never quite had time to do. It was a very rewarding exercise as I uncovered helpful things that I had long forgotten or thought I'd lost in earlier clear-outs. Thanks to my place on the staff side, I was kept up-to-date with notes and papers from many senior team meetings, which I would not otherwise have had access to. It helped to understand a bit of what was being planned because my manager was completely tied up in back-to-back Covid "silver" meetings and briefings.

In a phone call one afternoon, she described some of the areas of work where they were hoping to rede-ploy staff to work, including the Intensive Treatment Unit (ITU) and Occupational Health as well as Health and Safety. I was happy to offer my help in any of these areas, and a few days later, I was asked to join the Health and Safety team, which were tasked with rolling out "face-fit testing" of Covid protection masks. At a time, during lockdown, when people were limited to travelling no more than 5 miles from home, I found myself driving along the near-empty, beautiful scenery of the Highland road network, to a variety of community hospitals. It helped that the weather was glorious, but it felt very surreal in the context of such a dark time in so many peoples' lives. At least it meant that we could open the windows wide to let lots of fresh air circulate while we worked. I thoroughly enjoyed the whole experience of working with new people, in places where I had never visited before. There were still no Covid vaccines available so the risk of catching the virus was a very real and present danger to us all. Initially, we were given no protective gloves or masks ourselves, which was rather ironic in the context of a Health and Safety team... However, that changed after several weeks and we all travelled around as a group, ensuring that staff were confident about using the best-fitting face mask needed to protect them during their work. It was an important job and it kept me busy for several months in the summer of 2020. I managed to keep on top of other aspects of my job, although many of the usual meetings had been suspended, which helped. TEAMs' meetings became the norm and I noticed that they often allowed greater participation – both physically and in general communication — as people were better equipped to join in remotely and using the comments icons to share views or approval of the discussions. Face-to-face meetings had mostly taken place in Inverness before that, which made it a challenge to fully participate if it meant a 4-hour return journey or trying to connect via VC links. I think a lot of people enjoyed the voice that TEAMs gave them, so I hope that has continued. Participants were far more tolerant of each other's struggles to use technology and calls of "You're on mute!" were familiar to many. There were the inevitable funny moments, of course, when children who were home-schooling would walk behind a parent who was trying to contribute serious points in meetings held from a laptop on the kitchen table, to rummage through a cupboard or fridge for snacks. Cats would jump onto people's worktables and casually stroll across the keyboard, stopping to look down the camera or accidentally cutting off the connection. Occasionally, a tired parent would vent their annoyance at misbehaving children or animals, with expletive-filled language, only too late realising that they should have been on mute! As people became familiar with background settings, we could no longer examine their home décor, or contents of bookshelves, or even their selection of alcohol on the sideboard!

By September, the Scottish government had tasked health boards to set up Covid contact-tracing teams, led by public health consultants and advisors. There was inevitably a very tight deadline to get up and running and, after some initial, very hurried training. I became one of the senior NMAHPs to work in this role. We were a very varied group of health professionals — public health, AHP (me), and nursing — but we worked well together and enjoyed our temporary new roles. The essence of the team was to contact people who had been tested positive for Covid, in our area (NHS Highland), to gather details about their symptoms, recent contacts and daily routines. We then provided them with standard, national advice about self-isolation, keeping people around them safe and information about further sources of support or advice, if necessary.

We also had to call people with whom they had been in close contact, with much the same purpose. It gave us all a fascinating insight into the lives of people living, working in or visiting the Highlands. I was surprised at times to find myself calling people on the south coast of England, in rural Wales or Yorkshire, not to mention the contacts around Scotland. No workplace was out of limits either, and included people working in hospitality, military bases, emergency services, oil rigs, offices and schools, to list just a few.

For the most part, we were met with thanks from those we called, but not always. Some close contacts were angry and upset that they had to self-isolate and were not able to go to work — particularly those on zero-hours contracts. Others were furious, assuming that visitors had come to visit them even though they were already showing signs of Covid. Tearful young people longed to be home, being looked after by Mum and Dad, while they felt too ill to get out of bed. Others were in complete denial, of course, and quite resistant to following self-isolation advice, so we were sometimes on the receiving end of rants about conspiracy theories and challenges about our roles in it all. I sometimes found myself working 7 days a week, as I was still contracted to do my day job, so it became unsustainable in the longer term, and I stepped back from the team for a few months at the end of 2020 to focus on other things.

I very much missed the contact I had had with care home staff and residents, and I know that many of them wanted me to visit them. I wondered how our residents were coping being stuck, alone in their rooms, and how they were coping without seeing others. Social interaction has such a positive effect on our appetite, so there was a possibility that many would lose weight. However, I was able to continue to offer education and support remotely — initially via Zoom before TEAMs came along. I was also pleased, if maybe slightly daunted, to be invited by Prof Elaine Hunter to deliver webinars to national (across Scotland) and North of Scotland audiences. However, at the end of it all, I was proud to have been able to play so many varied roles in adapting to and delivering a professional Covid response. I may not have been working on the clinical front line in ITU (though I did offer), however, the work that the face-fit, testing and contact-tracing teams did was just as important. I wrote an article for "Dietetics Today", the BDA's monthly magazine, encouraging the dietetic workforce to recognise and celebrate the many transferrable skills that we have to offer as AHPs. The profession continues to develop into new areas of practice, and I look forward to seeing others come to recognise more fully and utilise the extensive skill set of dietetic colleagues.

Chapter 17— Retirement

Like many people, during 2020 and 2021, I started to reflect more on what really mattered to me — to live a good and fulfilling life. So many people had died – often alone without loved ones — or had lived and worked through extraordinarily stressful times. As we progressed through various Covid lockdowns and adapted to different ways of working and interacting with others, it occurred to me one week that life was too short and too fragile to remain doing what I'd always done. Young people today think nothing of taking time out to go travelling or change career at the drop of a hat. But I was from a student generation where we were expected to choose a profession, graduate and immediately start our working lives so I would never have dreamed of being anything other than a dietitian for decades to come. I still really enjoyed professional interactions and building networks with many national partners, working alongside care home staff and residents and writing in a variety of national journals, blogs and other formats. However, it occurred to me that I was coming up to the same age as my mother had been when she developed breast cancer, which severely affected her health and opportunities to enjoy her retirement as fully as she might have hoped. My husband and I had coped well together, in our little bubble, during the lockdown months. We often joked with others that we hadn't come close to killing each other, so it was easier to think more seriously about stepping away from the NHS and enjoying doing the things that we wanted to do more of together instead.

I took the opportunity of joining an on-line NHS pre-retirement course, which made me realise that, after more than 35 years' continuous service, I had both the means and opportunity to start afresh. At the end of June 2021, and with a degree of nervous apprehension, I duly gave 6 months' notice and took the opportunity of a 3-month phased retirement plan leading up to the end of the year. Although my final day at work was the 21st of December, my contract finally finished on the 31st — ready for a new life ahead from the 1st of January 2022.

I committed my time to planning something of a farewell training tour of care homes all around the beautiful North Coast 500 route, determined to leave with happy memories for me and for the social care staff and residents I worked with. I never tire of the beautiful scenery across the north of Scotland and often used to pinch myself, thinking that I was actually being paid to travel to homes in remote and rural areas. Driving to many parts of the Highlands, I enjoyed seeing the changing countryside during all the seasonal changes. It really is breath-taking at times and the wildlife can be quite distracting. One day, as I sat looking out at the beautiful view across Portree harbour eating my lunch, I had a bit of a lightbulb moment. I decided that I would celebrate the end of my career by reflecting on the positive highlights of my working life, in true dNMAHP style, using social media. In a nod to the "12 Days of Christmas", I worked my way through a 10-day version, posting highlights on each of my last 10 days at work. It was incredibly well received, and I was asked to write a final article for the Scottish government's AHPScot blog site to capture it all. Colleagues I hadn't heard from in years got in touch to tell me that they'd followed my career all this time, wishing me well and thanking me for all that I had done for them and our profession. Farewell messages came in from all the national partners I'd work closely with, as well as dietitians, AHPs, consultants and managers across the Highlands. It was lovely to re-connect and to remind myself of how far I had come since that first day at RGU in 1982. I am naturally a very positive person, but at times, I'd had the confidence knocked out of me. However, this process of letting go gave it back to me again in spades.

People kept asking me what I was planning next but all I wanted to do was spend a few special days at Christmas with my family and take time to decide what the future might look like. In the back of my mind, I had considered some other form of working with my dietetic hat: a training consultancy, freelance clinical work, more volunteering with the BDA maybe? I am thankful for the advice I got from an older friend who suggested that I wait 6 months and see how my life and priorities might have changed. Not long into my new life, I was still receiving retirement cards, flowers and gifts. However, I was especially delighted to receive a service recognition award, for my dedication and length of service to the profession, from the SDLN group. It was a nice way to finish my NHS career, to feel valued by peers across Scotland, and good to know that they thought that I had made a positive contribution to my profession.

It took quite a while to disengage from social media and looking at professional websites, still trying to keep up with news and developments just as I had at work. But gradually, the fog lifted and after enjoying several short holidays, the freedom to go walking, visiting places I'd never been and reading dozens of books, I realised that any form of future dietetic career would just interfere with my freedom to enjoy life! So, I put to bed all notions of practising and cancelled my HCPC subscription. It was a huge decision because, after 36 years, I was no longer able to call myself a dietitian (it is a protected title). I continued my BDA subscription as a retired member, but within the year, I had cancelled that too, feeling that much of what was being discussed had no relevance to my life "on the other side." It wasn't as hard a wrench as I'd thought, and I continued to observe from the sidelines using the power of social media feeds.

Life continues to surprise me, though, and in July 2023, I was delighted to receive a message from Dr Myra Mackenzie from RGU, informing me that the international journal of practice education had selected our article on the award-winning social care placements for dietetic students, to feature in their top-10 articles for a celebration tenth edition of the journal. We were humbled and delighted in equal measure as we prepared a short reflection of our work since it started in 2015. The retirement that just keeps on giving, eh?!

It's now almost two years since I stepped away from work in the NHS. I experienced an overwhelming feeling of freedom as I headed north from Inverness through the country lanes, with rock music playing loudly in the car. I can honestly say that I have never regretted my decision and can recommend retirement to anyone. Life is too short to keep waiting for life to happen, so embrace it while you have the opportunity and LIVE!

Chapter 18 — Reflections

The dietetic profession has changed beyond all recognition from the time that I started out all those years ago. New clinical technologies, application of research, health policy, the digital age and the willingness of colleagues, past and present, to stretch the boundaries of the role, have all been influential. We have gone full circle in the way we support people who need additional nutrition support. In my student days at Bristol, we could only offer homemade drinks. Pre-packaged drinks took over from the late 80s into the 2000s and we become almost totally dependent on them to care for people needing help to gain weight. We're now heading back to conventional ways of increased calorie and protein drinks. On the other hand, artificial tube feeding options — both feed and tubes — have given far greater flexibility and independence for patients and clinicians. When I think back to that one and only careers interview, I can smile, knowing how my instinct to study at RGU had been the best decision for me. I encourage teenagers, and others, to consider this as a career, given the variety of subjects studied and the evolving range of job opportunities that are available now; not to mention those that are still to emerge. Looking back on all my varied jobs, it's clear that most of the time, I've spent far more time helping people avoid losing weight than promoting weight loss. I've lost count of the number of times that I've told people what I did, only to hear the predictable "you'll have to give me a diet sheet" as they suck their stomachs in. The workforce profile and opportunities are now so much broader, and the skill mix gives so many more opportunities for staff to progress in their careers than ever before. The range of support staff at one end, and the expanding advanced practitioner posts at the other, offer so much diversity to any NHS team. The profession will continue to grow and expand into new areas of practice so I encourage students to remember that the start of their journey will undoubtedly reveal new opportunities over the horizon. It's great to see dietitians now being asked for expert opinion on news and in media channels. I'm hopeful that governments and other agencies will continue to appreciate the contribution, diversity and skills of dietitians in whatever role they have. The BDA and its membership will no doubt continue to keep promoting the unique expertise that they have and I look forward to a time when more dietitians are inspiring us with their transformational work "firsts".

So, after all that has gone before, would I change any of my decisions — maybe my choice of profession… my involvement with the BDA… all the moves around the country? The answer is a resounding no. I don't know where my path will take me next, but I have no regrets about the journey or in everything that I've experienced or achieved so far. I will always strive to give my best to whatever comes my way. I believe that things happen for a reason and that I would not be the person I am today without the many refining experiences and encounters that I've had along the way. It's been quite a rollercoaster ride at times — very squiggly, if you know what I mean. It's important to grow and learn from mistakes, and I'm no different from anyone else in that. Life's too short to look back regretfully or to stand still and stagnate. I've been able to take measured risks in many of the roles that I've had and choices that I've made. I have thrived on the opportunities to transform, innovate and improve both myself and the service areas I've worked in locally, nationally and internationally. As Winston Churchill famously said, "Success is not final, failure is not fatal: It is the courage to carry on that counts." In my many management evaluations over the years, I've been commended for my resilience and perseverance. My trophy cabinet is impressive but each award only reflects a moment in time. What got me out of bed each day at work was the opportunity to make a positive difference for patients and to share the experience with others; humbling as the honours, trophies or plaudits might be.

Writing this over the past two years has brought back so many great memories for me. Names of colleagues, patients and teams that I've worked with would suddenly come back to me in the middle of the night or when I was driving. Looking through my portfolios, old archives and emails at home also helped me remember some of the steps I've taken during my career. I have always kept positive messages, thank-you cards and complimentary emails from others, as a way of supporting my personal development and to strengthen my feelings of self-worth. This has helped me to remain confident and resilient during periods of great challenge or criticism. I would commend this approach to others, as it's far more objective and powerful to show someone else's view of your work or contribution than singing your own praises. To those colleagues who are already qualified, I encourage you to embrace the squiggle within you and take every chance to volunteer, accept invitations to speak, or write about your work. Always strive to make a difference — for patients, services, the profession and yourself. You never know where the most obscure encounter, development or opportunity will lead, so embrace change and you won't be disappointed. I hope that my varied insights and experiences will also help you to be courageous and try new things too.

Acknowledgements

I would like to take this opportunity to thank everyone who has inspired and supported me during my career. There are too many to mention but I've alluded to some in my reflections. I hope that I might have made a positive difference and inspired many colleagues and students too. Leaving a professional legacy is important to me but I couldn't have done it all, or written this account, without the encouragement and unconditional support of my immediate family and close friends. I hope this will be the first of several more books, which are still whirring around in my head.

Maybe reading my story will encourage others to do the same and enjoy their own trip down memory lane. Happy reflections!

Appendix I. Glossary of terms

A4C: Agenda for Change

AHP: Allied Health Profession

AIG: Action inquiry group

BAOT: British Association of Occupational Therapists

BBA: British Burns Association

BDA: British Dietetic Association

BOS: British Orthoptic Society

COHSE: Confederation Of Health Service Employees

CNO: Chief Nursing Officer

CPSM: Council for Professions Supplementary to Medicine (now the HCPC)

EFAD: European Federation of Dietetic Associations

DH: Department of Health

HCA: Hospital Caterers Association

HCPC: Health and Care Professions Council (previously Health Professions Council)

HMPS: His Majesty's Prison Service

IBA: Indian Burns Association

ICDA: International Confederation of Dietetic Associations

IR: Industrial Relations

ITU: Intensive Treatment Unit

JSCC: Joint Staff Consultative Committee

KSF: Knowledge and Skills Framework

MiP: Managers in Partnership

NALGO: National Association of Local Government Organisations

NES: NHS Education for Scotland

NHD: Network Health Digest

NMAHP: Nursing, Midwifery and Allied Health Professions (dNMAP – Digital NMAHP)

NOMS: National Offender Management Services

NPSA: National Patient Safety Agency

NUPE: National Union of Public Employees

PAMs: Professions Allied to Medicine

PCT: Primary Care Trust

PEAT: Patient Environment Action Team

PEC: Professional Executive Committee

PEG: Percutaneous Endoscopic Gastrostomy

PENG: Parenteral and Enteral Nutrition Group (BDA specialist interest group)

PT'A': Professional and Technical (committee of the Whitley Council)

RGU: Robert Gordon University

SoR: Society of Radiographers

TPN: Total Parenteral Nutrition

TUC: Trades Union Congress

References

MACKENZIE, M. and NEWMAN, E. 2017. Future proofing the dietetic profession*:* Exploring social care placements in pre-registration dietetic education. *International Journal of Practice-based Learning in Health and Social Care. Vol 5, no.1, pp.65-76.*